DISCARDED

smallpox

smallpox

The Fight to Eradicate a Global Scourge

David A. Koplow

CARL A. RUDISILL LIBRARY
LENOIR-RHYNE COLLEGE

UNIVERSITY OF CALIFORNIA PRESS

Berkeley / Los Angeles / London

RA
644
.S6
K675
2003
Apr 2004

University of California Press
Berkeley and Los Angeles, California
University of California Press, Ltd.
London, England
© 2003 by the Regents of the University of California

Library of Congress Cataloging-in-Publication Data
Koplow, David A., 1951–
    Smallpox : the fight to eradicate a global scourge / David A. Koplow.
        p.   cm.
    Includes bibliographical references and index.
    ISBN 0-520-23732-3 (cloth : alk. paper)
    1. Smallpox.   2. Smallpox—Prevention.   3. Smallpox—Epidemiology.
4. Smallpox—Cultures and culture media.   I. Title.
    [DNLM: 1. Smallpox—prevention & control—Russia.   2. Smallpox—
prevention & control—United States.   3. Health Policy—Russia.
4. Health Policy—United States.   5. International Cooperation—Russia.
6. International Cooperation—United States.   7. Variola virus—Russia.
8. Variola virus—United States.   WC 588 K83s 2003]
RA644.S6 K675   2003
616.9'12—dc21   2002005539

Manufactured in the United States of America
12   11   10   09   08   07   06   05   04   03
10   9   8   7   6   5   4   3   2   1

The paper used in this publication is both acid-free and totally chlorine-free
(TCF). It meets the minimum requirements of ANSI/NISO Z39.48–1992 (R 1997)
(*Permanence of Paper*).

To Pop
———

Contents

Acknowledgments

The author gratefully acknowledges the creative and energetic assistance of research assistants Amy Snell and Fred Lohr. At the University of California Press, Reed Malcolm and Cindy Wathen provided valuable assistance through the process of manuscript evaluation, and Erika Büky, along with Stacey Lynn and Harrison Shaffer of Green Sand Press, carefully brought the book through production. Thanks also to Sonya Manes for her excellent copyediting of the final manuscript.

INTRODUCTION

The virus responsible for smallpox—a tiny creature known as variola—has been a despised enemy of civilizations around the world. Over a period of at least three millennia it was second to none in inflicting human pain, suffering, and death. By some estimates, smallpox killed as many as 500 million people during the twentieth century alone, and as recently as thirty years ago, it was still at large in over thirty countries, attacking some fifteen million people annually and killing two million of them.

Through history, we have battled this foe with incantations, poultices, quarantines, and vaccinations. After struggling to contain it, we have at last conquered the disease globally and placed the last acknowledged vestiges of the virus in high-security confinement. Now, under the auspices of the United Nations, humans may be about to take a final, irreversible, step: to exterminate the last remaining captive samples of the smallpox virus. Thus, a quarter century after smallpox as a disease was wiped off the face of the earth, after additional years of painstaking struggle and research, the last two stockpiles of the causative virus (at least the last two that we know about)—stored in $1/2$-inch high plastic vials in $-70°$ Celsius liquid nitrogen baths inside secure isolation chambers at the Centers for Disease Control and Prevention in Atlanta, Georgia, and at the Russian State Research Center of Virology and Biotechnology near Novosibirsk—are targeted for destruction.

If activists in the World Health Organization and in many governmental and

1

private institutions around the world have their way, then within the next few years all the known variola samples, all the various strains, and all the residual infective materials will be inserted into an autoclave—a small, airtight laboratory sterilization furnace. The jets will be ignited, raising the temperature to 120° Celsius for forty-five minutes, and the process will be repeated. Then the vials that have housed the virus for so long will themselves be incinerated. In the end, there will be no tangible legacy at all of one of the most pernicious killers in earth's history.

We are thus on the precipice of a momentous decision: human beings are about to conduct the world's first *deliberate* extinction.

Extinction carries a certain irresistible cachet. The finality of eradicating not just a particular individual but an entire species arouses human curiosity and wonderment. The notion of permanently and deliberately divesting the planet of a discrete life form, whether a terrifying dinosaur or an elusive aquatic plant, is—as it should be—both humbling and awe inspiring.

Of course, extinctions occur all the time: the earth loses dozens, if not hundreds, of species every year, usually without public fanfare, often without even human cognizance. We lose flora and fauna we have rarely seen, hardly studied, and never cataloged. Many of these collective deaths, perhaps most, are at least partly attributable to human activity. We overhunt some species; we irrevocably destroy the critical habitats of others; pollution drives still more into the abyss. In some instances—dodo birds, carrier pigeons—the extinction has become a notorious case study for subsequent generations to abhor. In a few instances—bald eagles, snail darters—a monumental social enterprise has been launched to preserve the endangered species, occasionally becoming at least partially successful. In most instances, however, humans little note nor long remember the passage of a dying breed.

With the eradication of smallpox, however, human accountability for the destruction of another kind of creature becomes not only self-conscious but deliberate. This book is an analysis of that imminent, irrevocable action, investigating the facts underlying it, exploring the public values supporting it, and critiquing the decision-making apparatus leading up to it. The inquiry is necessarily both interdisciplinary and international in focus, examining the different categories of thought and activity that have led us to the brink of this decision. To understand our collective posture toward variola, and to think rationally about what to do next, we need to synthesize lessons from medicine, biology, military science, environmentalism, international organizations, and ethics. To decide whether to exercise the awesome power that technology and conscientious labor have now afforded us—and to decide what precedent to establish for the *next* time we are confronted with a comparable dilemma—we should pause now to deliberate a very delicate social choice.

In deciding whether to eradicate smallpox, the world community must address diverse and fundamental questions. Each of the next six chapters analyzes one key dimension of the story of smallpox. Chapter 1 scrutinizes the medical issues, beginning with a sketch of the history of smallpox and humankind's battle against it. It traces the devastating effects of smallpox across continents and through centuries. It also outlines the convoluted course of antismallpox activity, from ancient deity worship to Lady Montagu's eighteenth-century invocation of variolation, Edward Jenner's eighteenth-century discovery of vaccination, and Donald ("D. A.") Henderson's twentieth-century leadership of the dramatic and successful eradication campaign.

Chapter 2 then turns to the biological dimension, posing fundamental questions such as: What is a virus? Is it alive, as a distinct species? What might we learn from continued research on this creature—a pathogen that afflicts only human beings, with no known animal or plant reservoir? And what more could we do to protect ourselves against a future outbreak of it? The chapter also presents, in layperson's terms, an analysis of modern research into genetic engineering, surveying whether futuristic DNA-splicing techniques and cloning technology might have implications for variola preservation.

Next, chapter 3 considers the military dimension. It profiles how biological weapons agents, including the smallpox virus, have been conceptualized, and occasionally used, as weapons. Certainly disease has played a huge, albeit largely unintentional, role in hostilities: in virtually every international or internal conflict, more people (civilians and soldiers alike) have been felled by illness than by bullets or bombs. Pestilence has shifted battles, won wars, conquered empires, and changed history. However, most military authorities in the United States and elsewhere eventually came to dislike and distrust biological means of warfare, concluding that germs are simply too unpredictable and too uncontrollable for battlefield applications, and they were removed from most countries' active arsenals, unilaterally and voluntarily, more than two decades ago. Yet within the last few years, the revolution in genetic engineering has threatened to reverse that self-restraining judgment once again, and new incarnations of biological weaponry might prove to be far more effective and attractive—for terrorists no less than for regular armies. The upheavals on and after September 11, 2001, provide another fresh impetus for reexamination of the specter of unconventional warfare, such as smallpox bioterrorism.

The environmental dimension is the topic of chapter 4, which considers the extent to which the new, but increasingly entrenched, planetary regard for protection of biological diversity may inform the eradication decision. As we have come to appreciate the importance of husbanding our planet's scarce resources, we recognize the magnificent kaleidoscope of species—and their dazzling array of genetic variation—as carrying irreplaceable human value. Already legions of treaties, principles of customary international law, and domestic statutes constrain our heretofore clumsy disregard of other species. Even if these enactments turn out not to be legally binding on the novel question of preservation or destruction of a miniature creature such as a virus, they still exemplify important principles, values, and intellectual constructs that should inform our choices.

Chapter 5 discusses another, very different type of international institutional or organizational process issue: the role of the United Nations, specifically the World Health Organization (WHO), in deciding the fate of the smallpox virus. Who, in this world of independent, sovereign states and an increasingly dense thicket of amorphous multilateral nongovernmental organizations, has the legal authority to make the final decision for all humankind in this type of life-and-death matter? How has, and how should, the WHO bureaucracy and governing institutions engage this challenging issue, and what procedures should it employ in order to act wisely for us all?

Chapter 6 then confronts some of the profound ethical aspects of the smallpox eradication campaign. What social lesson will we teach future generations by our dealings with variola? What is the precedent we are establishing for the next time this type of deliberate extinction opportunity arises (which may not be far off)? What moral doctrines should we employ to evaluate whether the virus should be sustained? What substantive criteria are relevant to this type of determination, as humans, in a new way, opt to play God—or perhaps to play Dr. Frankenstein? These questions admit of no easy answers, but they must be asked and some irrevocable lines must be drawn.

To separate these distinct "dimensions" in this way is, admittedly, somewhat artificial. In this complex and unprecedented question, everything is connected to everything else, and the boundaries we have constructed between various intellectual disciplines are ill-defined and porous. Still, it may be useful to deconstruct the gnarled mass of issues that bear on this decision and tease out the identifiable strands for separate consideration.

The next two chapters shift gears a bit. Chapter 7 presents the case *for* extermination, marshaling the arguments in favor of destroying variola. It adduces five leading genres of arguments that can be asserted in support of the WHO's eradication decision, drawing freely upon the policy and technical considerations advanced in recent years by a variety of proponents. Chapter 8 presents the brief in opposition, assembling the best possible case *against* extermination. It weaves together five contrary arguments, again concentrating a variety of policies and preferences adduced by participants and observers. Together, these two presentations represent a scholarly and pragmatic debate drawing on all the preceding chapters, one that should help shape public policy dialogue.

Chapter 9 presents recommendations and concluding thoughts. My own "bottom line" is that I would *not* destroy these final exemplars of the smallpox virus. I would preserve them not out of a false sentimentality for a most undeserving scourge, nor simply out of an ethical concern that it is wrong for humans to play God in this way—although I take that to be a serious matter. Rather, I reject the hubris implicit in the conclusion that we no longer need the variola virus because our studies have already taught us everything we will ever need to know about it. I would retain these small reservoirs of DNA, just in case, as a relatively inexpensive form of biodiversity insurance, against the day when we may need this reprehensible scrap of genetic material to serve a noble end. Accompanying that conclusion are recommendations for the WHO, the United States, and other key actors on related policy matters ranging from counterterrorism initiatives to public health investments.

As far back as 1986, the WHO (or a cadre of experts within the institution) decreed that the variola residues should be promptly destroyed. Their target date was December 31, 1993—the first of a series of deadlines that have slipped unremarkably past while the virus samples linger on. The most recently established date (once described as the "final" extension for variola) was December 31, 2002—a day that has now been rendered moot, as have all the others, and will pass without dispositive action. The Bush administration has declared its opposition to any such destruction in the foreseeable future; its Russian counterparts have eagerly concurred; and the WHO bureaucracy, and its constituent member states, are still struggling to decide how to respond to the two dominant players' desertion from an erstwhile global consensus. No new target date for eradication has yet been established, but most WHO member countries still earnestly seek a prompt final resolution.

It is also important to note that the WHO may fail in any case to achieve its objective. Even if a strong global consensus is manifest, even if all countries declare their willingness to exterminate the last remaining variola samples, and even if the American and Russian repositories are, in fact, incinerated on schedule, all we can deal with in this way are the *known* stockpiles. All partisans acknowledge that other variola stashes may exist—hidden away by incompetence or malevolence—with the possibility of reemerging in some horrible scenario. Our policymaking, and our appreciation for the grand symbolism of our choices, must therefore be informed by that reality, and the rhetoric of our articulated goals modulated to that extent.

Stepping back just a bit, the variola question provides an opportunity to reflect anew that humankind has always struggled with, and against, nature, seeking to shield ourselves and our progeny from environmental threats. We have tamed rivers, felled forests, and established our dominion over the animals of the land and the fishes of the sea. We have waged ceaseless (but often fruitless) war against an array of biological pests: rodents, insects, and, now, viruses. But the step we contemplate taking with smallpox extends beyond merely resisting nature's forces, beyond domesticating a rival species or confining it to a circumscribed ecological niche. Here, we seek not only to control or defeat it; we intend to destroy it completely.

There is also a lesson here about risk. People have a difficult time thinking clearly and coherently about dangers that have a very low probability of occurrence but a very high cost if they do come about. Here, we are compelled to identify, assess, and trade off risks of very different types: bioterrorism, genetic engineering, laboratory accidents. How can we evaluate those risks in a manner that is rational, fair, and sensitive to all constituencies? In the main, the modern struggle against smallpox has been one of the finest achievements of the human race: we have demonstrated generosity, tenacity, inventiveness, and aplomb that have known no borders. In addressing the final step, the extinction of the last remaining viruses, how can that noble tradition best be sustained?

Over thousands of years the variola virus has tested our stamina, our intelligence, and our collective sensitivity. In struggling for a way to think coherently about this controversy, we have tended to fall back on familiar analogies, such as capital punishment: variola is depicted as an unrepentant convicted murder, now lingering on death row, with WHO considering whether to grant yet another stay of execution. That metaphor certainly has its appeal, but its explanatory power has limits, too. Now, we must face the reality that nothing in our collective experience is a valid model for organizing ourselves on this issue: it truly is a case of first impression. But just as surely, it will not be the last occasion for humans to confront these weighty issues.

CHAPTER 1

THE RISE AND FALL OF SMALLPOX

The medical history of smallpox is a saga of untold human suffering, unforeseen human inventiveness, and—ultimately—unprecedented human triumph. Smallpox was a loathsome disease, spreading around the world from antiquity to modern times. It was transmitted by an invisible virus; it infected an individual person and an entire community with remarkable speed; and it proved fatal to nearly one-third of its victims. Those who somehow survived a painful two-week period of fever, skin eruptions, and internal organ damage were usually left with severe scarring and sometimes blinded. There was no cure.[1]

ORIGINS OF THE DISEASE

No one knows for certain when, where, or how the smallpox virus first appeared on earth; we do know that it has circumnavigated the planet multiple times over many centuries, invading every place of human habitation. We also know more generally that the incidence of different forms of microbiological infection is probably almost as old as life itself: the first fossil traces of higher organisms, from half a billion years ago, reveal ample traces of insidious fungi and other parasitic attachments.

Even within written human history, it has proven impossible to trace the patterns of smallpox origins and evolution thoroughly, in part because of the lack, until the modern era, of a standardized medical lexicon. All sorts of plagues, rashes, pox diseases, and other pestilence were referred to interchangeably, and the ancient scribes' unscientific reports of the symptomatology do not always adequately distinguish the different types of ailments. Even in the modern era, accurate differential diagnosis has remained a challenge, as smallpox can sometimes masquerade as several distinct types of maladies, including the familiar chicken pox and more exotic novelties, until laboratory findings confirm the initial clinical impressions.

The image of smallpox as ubiquitous and ominous was well captured for the entire world by the British historian T. B. Macaulay in 1848: "Smallpox was always present, filling the churchyard with corpses, tormenting with constant fear all whom it had not yet stricken, leaving on those whose lives it spared the hideous traces of its power, turning the babe into a changeling at which the mother shuddered, and making the eyes and cheeks of the betrothed maiden objects of horror to the lover."[2]

The smallpox virus may have originated from a random mutation of some other, less venomous, and even older, strain of unknown virus, maybe around 10,000 B.C., perhaps somewhere in the fertile Ganges River plain in India. Some authors suggest—but it can be no more than speculation—that some relatively mild disease agents spontaneously adapted themselves from early domesticated animals or from lower primates to human hosts: the viruses that cause cowpox and monkey pox, for example, are still identifiable as close variola cousins today.

The term *variola* was derived in A.D. 570 by Bishop Marius of Avenches (near Lausanne, Switzerland) from the Latin *varius,* meaning spotted, or perhaps from another Latin term equally descriptive of the disease, *varus,* meaning pimple. In turn, the English word *smallpox* was coined in the sixteenth century, to distinguish between this disease and syphilis, which then became generally known as "the great pox," for the slight differences in the skin rashes the two maladies could produce. Other cultures likewise applied their own vocabulary in recognition of the power and destructiveness of smallpox: in some parts of West Africa, for example, it was known as *naba,* meaning "the chief of all diseases."

The first traces of what we now recognize as smallpox epidemics can be discerned among the records of ancient Egypt, India, China, and Greece, when agricultural settlements achieved population densities sufficient to sustain unbroken communication of the virus. Three mummies from the eighteenth and twentieth Egyptian dynasties (1570 to 1085 B.C.), for example, have exhibited the characteristic scarring interpreted by modern experts as evidence of smallpox. The first individually identified smallpox victim whose remains we can inspect, Pharaoh Ramses V, died in 1157 B.C., presumably from this disease: sophisticated modern analysis of his mummy has revealed the distinguishing pustular eruptions.[3] He thereby inaugurated a miserable tradition of fatal or near-fatal smallpox infection among royalty and prominent leaders, as well as legions of their followers, in a great many countries. By some estimates, 10 percent of all human deaths worldwide each year were attributable to this one illness.[4]

Some of the best evidence about ancient epidemics comes to us from war records: about 1350 B.C. the Hittite armies, for example, were devastated by a fatal contagious disease that apparently originated among the Egyptian prisoners of war they had seized in Syria. The illness killed their king, Suppiluliumas I, as well as his son and successor, Arnuwandas II, and led to a period of degenerative instability within the Hittite empire. Some experts familiar with the records now contend that this, too, was variola at work. Similarly, smallpox is credited with killing one-quarter of Athens's soldiers and countless civilians around 430 B.C., undermining that city-state in its competition with Sparta. Carthaginian troops also became infected with a contagious disease while besieging Syracuse in 395 B.C., depriving them of the potential for capturing Sicily and thereby threatening Rome; Alexander the Great's foot soldiers, while invading India in 327 B.C., likewise suffered from a virulent, often fatal, rash illness that may have been smallpox.

Half a world away, smallpox entered northern China in about 250 B.C. The Great Wall had been erected to repulse the invading Huns, but it proved little impediment to the virus they carried, and Chinese texts reported a terrible "epidemic throughout the empire" in 243 B.C. Japan, too, sparsely populated at that time to support endemic smallpox, was victimized nonetheless by recurrent epidemics, as visitors from China or elsewhere introduced the virus repeatedly, as early as the sixth century A.D.

On the average, smallpox killed at least 25 percent to 30 percent of the people it infected. The disease would spread with devastating speed, especially in the increasingly densely populated urban areas of Europe. Perhaps three to seven million people lost their lives to smallpox during the early days of the Roman Empire, and countless others were blinded or suffered other crippling impairments. Thereafter, increasing human mobility brought the disease to wider and wider areas of the planet, and sub-Saharan Africa, too, fell victim.

Through succeeding centuries, smallpox outbreaks occurred in an irregular geographic pattern. The only constant was the disease's ability to kill both the highborn and the commoner—not distinguishing between "princes and peasants," as the title of Donald Hopkins's 1983 book puts it. Queen Elizabeth I of England was infected in 1562; she survived, but two Japanese emperors, kings of Burma and Siam, and perhaps the Roman emperor Marcus Aurelius were less fortunate. Smallpox killed "a queen of England [Mary II], an Austrian emperor, a king of Spain, a tsar of Russia, a queen of Sweden, and a king of France in the eighty years before 1775."[5] Abraham Lincoln was stricken with a mild case of smallpox upon his return from delivering the Gettysburg Address in 1863; perhaps he acquired the virus from his youngest son, Tad, who also survived; the president probably passed the infection on to his valet, William H. Johnson, who died.

Four characteristics of smallpox shaped its transmission patterns. First, the disease was spread through relatively close contact: the virus can be propelled through the air for short distances or passed along by immediate physical contact with a diseased person or with his or her clothing or linens. Proximity was thus a requirement for dispersion. Second, smallpox appeared in an acute, manifest form; it could not be carried asymptomatically or secretly. Third, it virtually never struck the same person twice: anyone who contracted the disease and managed to survive it thereby incurred lifelong immunity. (Consequently, adolescents whose faces bore its characteristic pockmarks were much in demand as nannies and servants; anyone else could be a conduit for variola.) Fourth, the disease affected humans exclusively; there is no reservoir for variola in flora, fauna, soil, or air, as there is with so many other insidious disease agents.

The combination of those factors meant that smallpox would commonly appear in waves, several years apart. It might, for example, flare up in a particular city, where the closely spaced houses facilitated the virus's access to new bodies. A great many people could be quickly exposed to the disease. After the infection had run its course within the defined population, however, another outbreak was unlikely for several years, as most people would be either dead or immune. Only after a new generation had been born would there once again be a sufficiently large unprotected population for the virus to attack; when it was reintroduced, say, by a traveler, it would again work its way through the new victims. The grisly reality was that smallpox became, perforce, an episodic disease of children—in eighteenth-century Britain, for example, a full 90 percent of the victims were under ten years of age.[6]

A vivid illustration of the contagion was offered by the experience of the Spanish conquistadors in the New World in the early sixteenth century. Latin America, isolated from viral or other contact with Europe, was virgin territory for variola: no one there was already immune. When the virus was first imported into Caribbean islands by incoming slaves, whole tribes were instantly wiped out; half the native population of Puerto Rico was felled by smallpox within a few months in 1519. Later that year, when explorers Hernán Cortés and Panfilo de Narváez encountered the Aztec civilization of Mexico, variola accompanied them. As the disease spread quickly, the natives "died in heaps, like bedbugs."[7] The Spaniards, many of whom had survived smallpox epidemics as children, seemed impervious to the illness, a fact that heightened the impression that they had mystical powers. The Aztecs soon lost their emperor to smallpox, as well as numerous other local leaders who might have effectively resisted Cortés. Estimates of variola's death toll among the Aztecs range from two to fifteen million (out of a total population of less than thirty million), within only a few months.[8]

The macabre story was next repeated in Central America, as variola accompanied the Spanish southern advance upon the Mayan civilization. Epidemics struck Yucatan in 1520 or 1521, killing off half the population and a comparable percentage of its leadership. Likewise, the Incas in Peru were devastated a few years later, facilitating the ability of the small armies of Cortés and Francisco Pizarro to subdue opponents who greatly outnumbered them.

In North America, too, smallpox proved an essential, if unwitting, ally of the European colonizers. As late as 1600, there was probably no experience with smallpox north of Mexico, and, accordingly, no individual or social immunity. Following the earliest explorers, however, a decimating illness that may have been smallpox reportedly killed 90 percent of the Indians along the Massachusetts coast from 1617 to 1619. Another smallpox epidemic arose in the populations near Plymouth Colony in 1633, killing twenty immigrants from the *Mayflower* and whole tribes of Indians. Enormous epidemics soon swept westward, inflicting terror and mass death among tribes along the Great Lakes: the Hurons and the Iroquois were especially hard hit.

A century later, smallpox asserted itself again, during the French and Indian War of 1754 to 1763. In any particular battle, one side or the other (or both) suffered enormously from the illness, and neither could count on the ability to mount sustained military campaigns in the midst of disease. In 1755, the so-called Year of the Great Smallpox Epidemic, Native American tribes were profoundly struck, and thereafter outbreaks—at roughly one-decade intervals— plagued the cities of whites and villages of Indians alike.

During the Revolutionary War, smallpox altered military strategy and shifted the course of battles. George Washington (who himself had survived a bout with smallpox, caught during a visit to Barbados in 1751) was loath to send his troops into Boston in pursuit of a fleeing British General William Howe in 1776, because of a smallpox epidemic then raging in the city. Later, smallpox among the colonials (rather than the military prowess of British reinforcements) compelled them to break off their threatening siege of Quebec, which could have been a decisive rebel triumph. Smallpox continued to harass both sides for the duration of the war, and fear of the contagion even played a role in the logistical maneuvers leading up to the Yorktown campaign in 1781.

By the eighteenth century—when smallpox was killing an average of 400,000 people per year in Europe alone[9]—leading medical authorities in many countries had begun to differentiate smallpox from other, similar impairments and had developed a sophisticated understanding of variola's disease progression. With the increasing reliance on the scientific method, they had routinely and painstakingly recorded the progression of the illness in an individual and in an entire population. The inquiry was confounded, however, by the fact that the disease could assume markedly different characteristics in otherwise similar individuals, giving rise to nomenclature differentiating half a dozen different smallpox types, including "fulminating," "malignant," "benign," and "modified."

In a "standard" case, variola virus was thought to enter the human body through the lungs or, less frequently, the skin. Smallpox typically started with a ten- to fourteen-day incubation or latency period following the initial exposure (the "pre-eruptive stage"), during which the infected person exhibited no signs or symptoms of pathology. For the next three days (the "prodromal stage"), various flulike effects would emerge: some victims suffered headache, backache, nausea, fever, chills, convulsions, and delusions, and a scarlet rash might appear on the face or body. Then, oddly, for a day or two, the fever would subside and the victim would feel better, as if recovering from some other, less deadly, ailment.

At that point (the "eruptive stage"), however, the smallpox infection worsened. A rash would erupt and spread over the body, more densely on the face and extremities than on the torso. Gradually, the flat parts of the rash would rise into pimples, blisters, and, finally, pustules. Those would eventually dry into crusts or scabs. The skin would turn pink, then red, as if it had been burned or scalded; it felt hot to the touch and would sometimes peel off in limp sheets. Internally, the virus would invade the lungs, heart, liver, intestines, and other organs. Eyes were a particular target: ulceration of the cornea left about 1 percent of smallpox survivors blind in one or both eyes. For survivors, permanent scars on the skin, of widely varying number and intensity, were a characteristic legacy of the disease.

A victim might die within a few days after the onset of the intense symptoms or linger for two weeks or more. The immediate cause of death was usually either toxemia or a hemorrhaging into the skin, throat, lungs, intestines, or uterus. Potentially lethal secondary infections could also arise from opportunistic bacteria invading the lesions caused by the virus.

Communication of the illness to surrounding people was readily accomplished, particularly during the winter and spring. The skin rashes and the open sores on the throat were opportune conduits for the initial victim to expel millions of viruses into the immediate vicinity, where they could be inhaled by the next target. The period of infectivity could last three weeks, from just before the rash appeared until the last scab dropped off. (Fortunately, large outbreaks centered on schools or marketplaces were somewhat unusual: by the time a person was fully infective, he or she was usually bedridden. Families, and later, hospitals, became the virus's preferred venue for communication.) Corpses, too, could spread the virus, and a victim's clothing, sheets, towels, and shroud could retain dangerous pus or scabs, further accelerating variola's transmission. About half the people exposed to the virus—an event that could require only a few minutes' contact—would be infected by it, and a quarter to a third of those infected would soon perish.[10]

An important subsidiary mystery about smallpox concerns the birth of two new strains of the virus, closely related to the original smallpox agent but with noticeably different characteristics. Sometime during the late nineteenth century, a milder form of the disease, sometimes referred to as *amaas* or *alastrim*, was identified in Southern Africa and the West Indies: it generally caused less severe pockmarking, and was fatal in only about 1 percent of cases. Subsequent laboratory analysis confirmed that this new agent, eventually designated *Variola minor*, was genetically distinct from, although quite similar to, the original breed, which then became known as *Variola major*. Infection with either strain resulted in cross-immunity: anyone who survived a bout with one could not be infected by the other.

As *Variola minor* spread through Brazil, England, and especially North America, it tended to displace its more vicious cousin, and local fatality rates declined precipitously. To compound the oddity, a third, intermediate strain was uncovered in East and West Africa in 1963: *Variola intermedius* killed about 12 percent of its victims.[11] To this day, no one knows where, when, or how these less noxious smallpox relatives crept into existence.

TREATMENT REGIMENS

The horrors of smallpox inspired a wide variety of creative treatment regimens, derived in each age from the prevailing social misunderstandings of the nature and origins of diseases. Many early civilizations, in India, China, Africa, and Latin America, designated a god or goddess of smallpox and offered sacrifices to honor or appease the deity. Others routinely practiced therapeutic bleeding, to leach the body of "excessive humors" and restore the internal balance that could ward off contagion. "Heat therapy" was the leading treatment in sixteenth-century Europe, although it is now considered inapposite to deal with a fever by packing the victim in blankets and huddling next to a fire. Some cultures, overresponding to the color of the smallpox rash, adopted "red therapy": surround the diseased individual with red-colored blankets, curtains, and other items, have him or her drink red liquids, and use only red implements in treatments. As silly (or even dangerous) as some of those approaches now seem, modern medical science has been able to do little better. Even today, there is no specific treatment for smallpox, and there is no effective antiviral medication; a case of smallpox generally still must run its course.

As the transmission mechanisms of smallpox and other diseases became more obvious, efforts at isolation and quarantine became common. Ships arriving from distant ports were sometimes carefully inspected before crew and cargo could disembark, and sick passengers were segregated from the community at large. Townspeople tried to avoid, or even to expel, smallpox-infected individuals from their midst, hoping to cut short the disease cycle. But inconsistent enforcement of these rules often rendered futile the primitive public health measures.

The first efficacious medical process for combating smallpox was "variolation" (or "inoculation"), which amounted to deliberately inducing a mild form of the disease, in the hope that the victim would recover and thereby gain lifelong immunity. Ancient Chinese, Indian, and African cultures had performed this process for centuries, following a variety of treatment regimens. In China, a dried powder composed of smallpox skin crusts harvested from a current disease victim was inhaled by others, like taking snuff. In the Middle East, a small amount of pus from a smallpox lesion was inserted into a cut on the arm of the person to be protected.

An individual who acquired smallpox artificially in this fashion would ordinarily suffer a moderate case of the disease—less rash, shorter illness, and only about a 1 or 2 percent chance of dying.[12] (But he or she was still fully infectious and could spread full-strength smallpox to other people.)

A few European authorities had become generally familiar with the concept and practice of variolation, but the medical establishment there proved too conservative to consider seriously the potential of the process. Variolation failed to gain widespread attention and acceptance in the West until it was aggressively promoted by Lady Mary Wortley Montagu, whose husband was the British ambassador to the Ottoman Empire from 1717 to 1718. After observing the technique's effectiveness among the Turks and having her own two children successfully variolated, she sponsored the concept at home. During the smallpox epidemic of 1721, two daughters of the Prince of Wales (the future King George II) were variolated, too, thereby ensuring the procedure's notoriety, if not its immediate acceptance, throughout the country.

At about the same time, variolation arose in the American colonies, as the Reverend Cotton Mather in Boston learned of the practice from his African slave, Onesimus. Mather, too, promoted it within the local medical community during a 1721 smallpox outbreak. He and his associates, however, encountered considerable resistance, both from other physicians and the citizenry, who feared that variolation could become a vehicle for inadvertently spreading the disease even more widely. There was also a popular sentiment against any activity that would interfere with the "natural" course of smallpox. Mather and his "progressive" associates were condemned for ungodly hubris and became a target of verbal and physical brickbats.

Many of the American colonies passed laws to prohibit or tightly regulate variolation; because of this legislation, the practice was much less common in America than it became in England. One ramification of that difference was that early in the Revolutionary War, British soldiers were noticeably less susceptible to the threat of smallpox. George Washington, whose face was deeply pitted as a result of his own bout with smallpox at age nineteen, was initially an outspoken opponent of variolation, believing it would spread the disease. Upon learning of a supposed British plot to use smallpox as a weapon against the Continental Army, however, he assembled a special unit of one thousand pockmarked fighters to counteract the danger that the Redcoats might pose. Shortly thereafter, Washington became a zealous convert to variolation, and in 1777 he ordered compulsory variolation of all new recruits.

The next achievement in the struggle against smallpox came from Dr. Edward Jenner, a rural English physician who had come to practice variolation routinely and who, himself, had almost died as a result of variolation when he was eight years old. He observed that dairymaids who had been infected with a mild pustular skin infection known as cowpox were thereafter confident that they could never be stricken with smallpox, and the local experience (or, at least, the folklore) seemed to corroborate the connection. After a decade of theorizing and empirical observation, Jenner undertook his famous experiment on May 14, 1796, injecting eight-year-old James Phipps of Berkeley with cowpox pus obtained from lesions on the hand of a milkmaid named Sarah Nelmes. When later Phipps turned out to have robust immunity against smallpox variolation attempts, Jenner published his thesis and recommendations.

Jenner's proposals, like Montagu's and Mather's, stimulated strong reactions:

both profound celebrations for salvation from smallpox, and intense, sporadic opposition for promoting an allegedly unnatural and dangerous deviation from established medical practice. But the value of Jenner's innovation soon became obvious, and the practice rapidly spread throughout the world. The difficulties of transoceanic conveyance of the infective cowpox material to waiting doctors across the Atlantic and elsewhere were overcome by impregnating threads with dried vaccine, or by maintaining an unbroken chain of arm-to-arm serial infection among ship passengers throughout the weeks of the voyage.

Because the original infective material was derived from cowpox, Jenner labeled his process "vaccination" (after the Latin *vacca,* cow). To memorialize that innovation, Louis Pasteur in 1881 generalized the term *vaccination* to apply to all other sorts of immunizing injections, including those for other illnesses. Today, we recognize the cowpox virus as a separate species but a close familial relative of the smallpox virus , even though we do not fully understand the operational principles of cross-immunity.

But another mystery remains. The virus that has been used over a period of several decades to vaccinate against smallpox—all the various strains employed throughout the United States and the world —is no longer true cowpox. The modern prophylactic, known as *vaccinia virus,* is a novel, separate creature. It may be a hybrid, the result of a microscopic mutation that somehow combined some of the features of the germs causing smallpox with those of Jenner's cowpox, and perhaps with those of yet another related disease known as "horse pox." In the two hundred years since Jenner, at some unknown time and place, the original stocks of cowpox virus that were used for vaccination have all been replaced with vaccinia virus, which has proven to be more effective and robust in producing immunity. Remarkably, that transformation to the "new" protective strand of orthopox virus was somehow inadvertent, invisible to the practitioners, and global.

As great a boon to humankind as the smallpox vaccination was, however, it was not a panacea. First there were risks of side effects: about one person in fifty thousand would experience adverse reactions of various sorts, and about one in a million would die. Other unfortunate people would inadvertently acquire other viral or bacterial infections along with the intended vaccination, and still others presented special conditions that contraindicated use of the vaccine altogether.[13] Moreover, the vaccination did not confer *lifelong* immunity, the way that variolation (or exposure to a full case of smallpox) did: after about ten years, a repeat was necessary. Also, many self-advertised vaccinators were dishonest, careless, or incompetent, or they dealt with impure or impotent vaccine strains, so in some areas, large numbers of the putative vaccinations were ineffective. In addition, many people, in many countries, continued to deride the whole concept of vaccination (especially compulsory vaccination) as immoral, an interference in the natural order of life, or an infringement upon personal autonomy. And, as with any medical procedure, financial and logistical barriers impeded the effort to vaccinate all those in need.

Consequently, smallpox persisted, and in some places thrived, around the world. Three major European pandemics, in 1824–1829, 1837–1840, and 1870–1875, spread the disease throughout the continent—not with the same virulence of earlier centuries, but deadly nonetheless. Russia suffered 100,000 smallpox deaths in 1856; France between 60,000 and 90,000 in 1870–1871; and Germany 162,000 in 1871–1872.[14]

Into the twentieth century, smallpox remained a global scourge—it was endemic in 124 countries in 1920—but it was no longer universal. Germany and the Scandinavian countries had reduced smallpox deaths to small numbers through compulsory vaccination, although European Russia still lost over 400,000 people to smallpox during the period 1900 to 1910, and Spain and Italy were hit hard, too. In the United States (a country reluctant to adopt mandatory antismallpox measures), an outbreak of a mild form of smallpox infected 130,000 people from 1901 to 1902 and 200,000 in 1920 to 1921. Some 64,000 Filipinos perished from smallpox from 1918 to 1919; India regularly reported over 100,000 smallpox fatalities per year; and Nigeria suffered 22,000 cases, including 6,000 fatalities, in 1930.[15]

Even after World War II, when endemic smallpox had been eradicated from most of the developed countries, it was more out of sight than out of mind. Thousands of cases were still being reported annually around the globe, and perhaps only 1 percent of the cases were accurately tabulated. Massive, sometimes deliberate, underreporting was the norm, concealing what were probably fifty million cases of smallpox per year in the 1950s.[16] Accordingly, compulsory vaccination of the population continued in many countries, international travelers were watched closely, and episodic eruptions of the disease were endured with alarming frequency.

For example, in 1945, an American soldier returning from Japan ignited an outbreak of sixty-five cases (twenty of them fatal) in Seattle, Washington.[17] The last eruption of the disease in the United States occurred in 1949, when eight people were infected (with one death) in the lower Rio Grande valley of Texas, but smallpox scares or rumors were persistent thereafter.[18] Other countries, industrialized and nonindustrialized alike, continued to import smallpox episodically into the 1970s—there were forty-nine reintroductions of the disease into Europe between 1950 and 1971—often with widespread fatalities and panic.[19]

As late as 1967, cases of smallpox were still being reported in forty-four countries, and the disease was considered endemic in thirty-one countries, containing some 60 percent of the world's population. There may have been as many as ten to fifteen million cases that year, resulting in some two million deaths.[20] The disease that had originally afflicted all of humankind had, by this point, evolved essentially into a problem of the poor: less developed countries south of the equator were continuously devastated, while the economically developed countries had managed, more or less, to barricade themselves against the worst effects of variola.

THE GLOBAL ERADICATION PROGRAM

The idea of developing a worldwide campaign to eradicate smallpox flickered hopefully from the first moments of Jenner's discovery. Farsighted people immediately waxed rhetorical about wiping out the disease and freeing humankind from its burden. As Thomas Jefferson wrote to Jenner in 1806, "You have erased from the calendar of human afflictions one of its greatest. Yours is the comfortable reflection that mankind can never forget that you have lived. Future nations will know by history only that the loathsome smallpox has existed."[21] However, more than a century and a half were to pass before concrete collective steps were taken.

With such virulent diseases, of course, any local solutions remain imperfect—no population could be secure from the threat of smallpox, as long as the disease retained its foothold anywhere—especially as human mobility dramatically increased. At the same time, many people disputed the notion that complete eradication (as opposed to containment and management of the disease) would ever be universally possible. Still, piecemeal progress was achieved, and smallpox was increasingly erased from the developed world during the twentieth century.

Public attention—driven by both humanitarianism and a cost-effective self-interest—turned increasingly to cooperative efforts at developing a worldwide solution. Eventually, global health authorities were able to demonstrate convincingly that the financial costs to the developed countries of sponsoring an effective universal smallpox eradication campaign would be more than offset by releasing themselves from the recurrent national costs of smallpox prevention and monitoring.

In 1950, the Pan American Sanitary Organization (a forerunner of the Western Hemisphere's arm of the World Health Organization [WHO], which was itself a "specialized agency" of the then new United Nations) approved a program to eradicate smallpox from the Americas. Within only eight years, and at a cost of less than $75,000 annually, that goal was accomplished for the Caribbean, Central America, and much of South America, although not for Brazil or Argentina.[22] In 1958, at the annual World Health Assembly meeting in Minneapolis, Victor M. Zhdanov of the Soviet Union further proposed, and the WHO then adopted as its official policy, the principle of seeking global smallpox eradication. This was a bold, unprecedented bureaucratic move, and in the face of technological, financial, and logistical limitations, it soon foundered. Competition with other diseases was undoubtedly an inhibiting factor: many countries were more concerned with malaria or measles, for example, than with smallpox, and it was difficult to craft a single-minded organizational approach.[23]

In January 1967, the WHO mandate was renewed, under the aegis of the Intensified Smallpox Eradication Program (ISEP), this time with a modest pot of $2.4 million in seed money, and a ten-year time frame to concentrate the energies.[24] Dr. Donald ("D. A.") Henderson, a medical epidemiologist on detail from the U.S. Public Health Service, assumed leadership of the WHO campaign and immediately set about creating the necessary infrastructure, including a multinational cadre of talented and dedicated individuals.

Immediate ISEP goals were improvement in the international mechanism for identifying and reporting smallpox cases (99 percent of which were estimated not to have made it into published national statistics) and in the development and mass production of unprecedented quantities of high-quality freeze-dried vaccine. (The Soviet Union alone donated nearly 1.4 billion doses of vaccine to the antismallpox campaigns.) Extraordinary inventiveness also came to the rescue, with both high technology (the jet injector, capable of vaccinating up to 1,000–1,500 people per hour) and low technology (the bifurcated needle, easily sterilized for repeated uses, not requiring any spare parts or maintenance, and simple to train nonexperts to use in the field).[25]

Political factors exerted influence as well. In the first instance, leadership by the planet's two superpowers, the United States and the Soviet Union, was essential in crafting and sustaining the global enterprise. Scores of countries temporarily set aside some of their usual insistence on rigid sovereign autonomy to collaborate in a remarkably open and accommodating fashion; seventy-nine nations tolerated a degree of foreign expert intervention that had not always been so graciously accepted in other contexts. At the same time, the WHO program had to surmount ten years of global political sensitivities, civil wars, apartheid, and strained relations, all during some of the darkest days of the cold war.

West and Central Africa were among the first targets of the Intensified Smallpox Eradication Program, selected to demonstrate that WHO efforts could succeed even in countries with systemic poverty and starkly limited domestic health infrastructures. An early strategic breakthrough was the adoption of the "surveillance-containment" concept: instead of seeking to vaccinate *everyone* (i.e., attempting to achieve a near 100 percent compliance record in each country), a less ambitious but equally successful tactic was to reliably identify and locate each new smallpox outbreak and for each of these locales immediately vaccinate everyone who may have already, or still might, come into contact with the virus. Quarantining an area and sealing off the outbreak before the virus could spread very far proved more manageable than the Herculean task of vaccinating truly everyone.

Twenty countries in West Africa (including six of those previously identified as among the most highly endemic smallpox locales in the world) were declared to be smallpox free within three and one-half years of the campaign's initiation. Other successes followed: Brazil encountered its last smallpox case in April 1971,

Indonesia in January 1972. By the end of that year, variola's formerly global range had been restricted to six countries: India, Pakistan, Bangladesh, Nepal, Ethiopia, and Sudan.

This record of swift success should not suggest that the outcome was easy or foreordained. Indeed, civil wars and international armed conflicts disrupted the program; political interference was a constant worry; harsh temperatures, monsoons, and other local conditions impeded the efforts of the UN officials; resources were always scarce; and resistance from skeptical, disorganized, dishonest, or fearful natives was common. In some circumstances, WHO representatives had to walk miles, lugging their equipment to remote villages where pox illnesses had been fragmentarily reported, and undertake often fruitless house-to-house searches for the elusive variola. The virus would occasionally skip "behind the lines," suddenly reappearing in West Germany in 1970, in Yugoslavia in 1972, or in other locations where it had seemingly been eradicated much earlier. Even massive tragedies were not yet a thing of the past: as late as 1974, a terrible smallpox epidemic in northeast India killed 25,000 people.[26]

But the WHO program persisted, eventually eliminating even the final variola bastions. The last known case of naturally occurring smallpox was found in Somalia (ironically, a country that had been smallpox free for over a decade but where importation from Ethiopia had reestablished the disease) in October 1977. Ali Maow Maalin, a twenty-three-year-old cook in a hospital in the coastal town of Merka, had occasionally volunteered as an aide to the WHO workers, although, oddly, he himself had never been vaccinated. He developed the characteristic rash shortly after accompanying a smallpox victim to a vaccination site. His case was quickly identified, additional vaccinations were given to all his associates, and he soon recovered fully. No one else—in Somalia, or elsewhere around the world—has since suffered from endemic smallpox.

The standards and practices of the WHO required two years of disease-free conditions before a country could be officially declared rid of smallpox. During those intervals, the vaccination campaigns continued, and efforts intensified to identify any remaining possible eruptions—including offering up to $1,000 to anyone who could produce another case. Even suspect cases were treated as international emergencies, prompting painstaking investigation and analysis. Unless the WHO certification regime was, and was perceived as being, airtight, national authorities would not rely upon it, and they would still be reluctant to relax their vaccination efforts and other antismallpox activities. Finally, on December 9, 1979, the crowning moment came: the United Nations campaign ceremoniously certified that the world was free from the disease.

Even as smallpox was being eradicated in the world at large, however, samples of variola virus remained plentiful in laboratories. Some of these strains were held for research purposes, some were kept as exemplars to help forensic experts identify any newly emergent virus strains, and some were apparently maintained due to simple bureaucratic inertia. The quality of the labs that housed the stockpiles varied enormously, as did their safety procedures and research protocols. In 1975, at least seventy-five laboratories, dispersed all over the planet, held infective variola stocks. Upon prompting by the WHO, many of these institutions consented to destroy their repositories or ship them to central collections, so by 1977 only eighteen reported retention of the virus, and that number gradually declined to only two by 1983.[27]

One factor spurring the countries to destroy or consolidate their smallpox virus stocks was the hazard posed by variola—as vividly illustrated by two infamous British laboratory accidents. The first, in London in March 1973, occurred when Ann Algeo, a twenty-three-year-old unvaccinated technician at the Mycological Reference Laboratory at the London School of Hygiene and Tropical Medicine casually observed a (presumably vaccinated) coworker harvest (on an open workbench in the lab) some variola samples that had been grown in eggs for research purposes. The observer became ill and was hospitalized with what was later identified as a mild case of smallpox—but the diagnosis was not timely, and she stayed in a general hospital ward for a week. During that time, she passed the infection to two unsuspecting people who had come to visit a relative in an adjacent bed, and they became the first smallpox fatalities in Britain in over a decade. A nurse who cared for one of those two victims was also infected, but she managed to recover.

Five years later, an even more peculiar laboratory anomaly occurred in Birmingham, England. Janet Parker, a forty-year-old medical photographer, worked in a small office and darkroom located one floor above the Department of Medical Microbiology laboratory of the University of Birmingham, where smallpox research was conducted without what we would now insist on as fundamental safety standards. In August 1978—nearly a year after the last "natural" smallpox case in Somalia—she became fatally ill with the disease. Post-mortem investigators speculated that the virus may have worked its way upward, through a ventilation and service duct, to a small telephone booth that Parker had occasionally used; alternatively, she may have had face-to-face contact with laboratory personnel or visitors.

In any event, Parker (who had last been vaccinated twelve years earlier) died within a month of infection, but before being hospitalized, she came into contact with a great many unsuspecting people—three hundred of whom were identified, tracked down, vaccinated, quarantined, and monitored. Only one of these three hundred, her mother, acquired the illness—fortunately, a relatively minor case. Two other deaths occurred as a result of the stresses of the outbreak. Parker's father, presumably strained by the chain of events, suffered a heart attack and died after visiting his daughter in the hospital. And Professor Henry Bedson, a world-famous scholar on smallpox, and the director of the Birmingham laboratory whose faulty procedures had initiated the outbreak, shortly thereafter committed suicide while quarantined at his home, ridden by guilt and distraught that he had misled British and WHO authorities about his laboratory's procedures, intentions, and safeguards.

These laboratory accidents sound a cautionary note, not simply about maintaining adequate safeguards and rigorous housekeeping procedures but also about the potential social consequences of a major mishap: if variola were somehow to escape today, the consequences for the world could be profound. Unlike in earlier generations, there is little natural immunity left in the world—the vast majority of the human population has not been recently vaccinated, and only a small percentage are now veterans of the disease. Through most of human experience, most outbreaks of smallpox had some "natural" limit: when the virus had exhausted the younger generation, butting up against those who had acquired immunity during an earlier epidemic, it died out. Today, however, the situation for humans globally is more akin to that of the seventeenth-century Native American tribes, who were devastated by their initial exposure, because none of their members had immunity. Like them, the global population today once again approaches 100 percent vulnerability.

An important difference is the existence today of a known and reliable vaccine. The world resolved in 1980 to maintain a security stockpile of heat-stable, freeze-dried vaccinia, with 200 million doses to be held by the World Health

Organization and another 100 million in various national stocks. The WHO inventory was to be preserved in appropriately cold storage (−20° Celsius), in two sites, Geneva, Switzerland, and New Delhi, India, and was supplemented by a stash of about 3.7 million bifurcated needles, as well as by reliable seed lots capable of producing more serum, should the need arise.[28]

Relatively soon, however, those "safety net" plans were frustrated. Difficulties maintaining proper quality control and funding the contemplated standby stockpiles led to reductions in the inventory and its consolidation in Switzerland. Production of new vaccine virtually stopped, and the capacity to generate additional vaccinia atrophied. In 1986, the relevant WHO committee determined that continued maintenance of the global inventory was no longer necessary, and the current WHO stockpile amounts to no more than 500,000 doses.[29] National holdings in various countries may now total about sixty to ninety million doses of uneven quality.[30]

Through 2001, the United States housed a ready stockpile of six to fifteen million doses of vaccinia, enough for no more than about 6 percent of the national population.[31] Questions have arisen regarding the continuing viability of these aging stocks—U.S. manufacture stopped in 1975—and some deterioration due to time and moisture has undoubtedly occurred. Still, governmental authorities not only deem the vaccine sufficiently potent but have considered the possibility that if a need ever arose, the vaccine could be diluted perhaps five or tenfold, allowing treatment of millions more people.

In addition, the U.S. government has recently launched no fewer than three programs to produce additional smallpox vaccine.[32] First, the Department of Defense, through its Joint Vaccine Acquisition Program, contracted in 1997 with a Maryland firm called BioReliance to deliver 300,000 doses of an improved vaccine for $22.4 million (approximately $70 per dose). This inventory, to be administered under the Smallpox Vaccine Biodefense Program to service members deployed to the locations of greatest threat, would consist of essentially the traditional vaccinia virus, but it would be manufactured with improved, cleaner and safer, techniques still to be developed and tested.[33]

Second, the Centers for Disease Control and Prevention (under the U.S. Department of Health and Human Services) in 2000 awarded a $343 million contract to OraVax, a Massachusetts biotechnology company, to manufacture forty million doses of vaccine beginning in 2004 and continuing through 2020 for a stockpile for the general civilian population at a cost of about $8 per dose.[34] The quantity of forty million was based on the recommendations of the Working Group on Civilian Biodefense, but after the October 2001 anthrax scares, and amidst increasing concerns about bioterrorism generally, both the quantity and the delivery timetable were modified.[35]

For both these contracts, the process of obtaining (or somehow obviating) approval from the U.S. Food and Drug Administration—an institution that rigorously regulates the marketing of new pharmaceuticals—may prove to be daunting. Although the vaccinia virus itself remains essentially the same as it has been for decades, the process for generating and collecting it in quantity must now be modernized. The traditional technique had been to obtain pus from the pox lesions on the flank tissues of an infected calf, but that method, of course, also harvested a plethora of unwanted bacteria and other contaminants. Modern laboratory techniques to ensure sterile preparations, now mandatory for any new pharmaceutical substances, would require careful development and FDA certification, which can require expensive and time-consuming testing. The FDA has pledged to intensify its review of any new smallpox vaccine production and has promulgated flexible new regulations to streamline the process in these extraordinary situations, but the agency cannot become merely a "rubber stamp" where drug safety and efficacy are concerned.

Third, following the September 11, 2001, terrorist attacks on the World Trade Center and the Pentagon, the Bush administration announced plans to seek $500 million in emergency funds to procure 300 million doses of smallpox vaccine—enough to treat everyone in America—by the end of 2002. Disputes over the contracting process and feuds between small and large potential bidders threatened to disrupt the process, but an immense quantity of new vaccine was scheduled for prompt delivery.

Two propitious developments then intervened. First, experiments confirmed that the existing vaccine stocks could be diluted at least five times and still retain their effectiveness—suddenly multiplying the available protections. Second, Aventis Pasteur, a French vaccine-making company, discovered a previously overlooked inventory of eighty-five million doses of similar vaccine, housed in its Pennsylvania warehouse, and donated it to the U.S. government. Suddenly, the prior shortage of smallpox vaccine was transformed into an oversupply, and other countries, too, were pursuing the manufacture of additional stocks.

No government currently intends to resume universal vaccination of civilian populations, and it is not clear whether the antismallpox treatment would be made available for individuals who sought it (as some already have).

Along with building up an immense vaccine inventory, there must be an understanding of the vaccine's limitations. Vaccinia is strongly contraindicated for many people: those with skin diseases such as eczema, those immunosuppressed by diseases (such as HIV/AIDS) or by organ transplants, pregnant women, and others. Statistically, the record has been that slightly more than one person in one million has died due to adverse vaccine reactions, and many more have been incapacitated for short or long periods. The frequency of serious complications from vaccinia was higher than that for any other vaccine now on the market to combat any other disease. Current projections have raised fears that a nationwide smallpox vaccination campaign today might result in as many as 600 to 1,000 deaths.[36]

Moreover, the most suitable medication to combat these often unforeseeable cases of encephalitis or other dangerous conditions, a substance known as vaccinia immune globulin (VIG), is exceedingly rare. The government's stockpile has grown so small—only 675 doses are now available—that virtually all smallpox vaccinations have long been suspended. Efforts to generate more VIG are also under way, but the process is laborious.[37]

As a result of the risk of severe adverse reactions, the World Health Organization has reaffirmed its conclusion that mass vaccination of civilians, in the absence of evidence of a smallpox outbreak, is not warranted. The traditional surveillance and containment strategy, developed and perfected during the global smallpox eradication campaign—of quickly identifying and isolating any cases, shipping vaccine stocks to the affected area immediately, and vaccinating all the potentially exposed people—would be used instead.[38]

Worldwide health security may therefore not be as perilous as it might seem, even should variola manage to "escape." Nevertheless, the adequacy of that safety net is now being questioned, and one of the ironies arising from humankind's successful battle against smallpox is that our guard has been let down, and our "herd immunity" has largely expired. As many as 120 million

Americans have never been vaccinated against smallpox and are fully vulnerable. The protection that older Americans once enjoyed from previous vaccinations has surely waned, at an unknown rate—no one really knows how rapidly the vaccine protection declines (either in the sense of avoiding the disease altogether or in suffering only a relatively modest version of it). As a result, any smallpox incidents now could carry enormous adverse potential.

The world has been free from the smallpox disease for over twenty years. In 1971, the U.S. Public Health Service recommended termination of the long-standing program of routine vaccination of civilian populations in this country, and that alteration in state and local practice became the norm within a few years. In 1982, the WHO's international health regulations deleted smallpox from the list of vaccinations required for international travel, and most countries followed suit. In 1983, Wyeth Laboratories, the only licensed producer of smallpox vaccine in the United States, discontinued the general distribution of the vaccine. By 1986, routine vaccination had ceased in all countries. The termination of these ambitious vaccination programs, and of the associated quarantine procedures, was an enormous boon for the affected countries— they saved far more in foregone protection costs than they had contributed to the WHO smallpox eradication campaign. In financial terms, then, apart from mitigating human suffering, the eradication effort was a monumental success.[39]

In the United States, by the early 1980s, only military personnel and poxvirus researchers continued to receive automatic protection against variola. North Atlantic Treaty Organization countries, including the United States, as well as Israel, Australia, Sweden, and a few others, persisted in vaccinating all or most troops. The Soviet Union had halted smallpox vaccination even for its soldiers in 1979 but resumed the practice in 1984, apparently in part because the United States had continued the immunization program for its military. In 1990, the United States terminated the program of automatic smallpox vaccination of service members—a decision driven more by concerns about adverse side effects than by the ending of the cold war. Russia, Canada, and others stopped shortly thereafter (although some special forces elements may still receive this form of protection), and only Israel is known to continue routine military vaccination on a large scale today.

The last remaining ampules containing the variola virus (at least the last specimens that the world knows about) have now been concentrated in two freezers. The Centers for Disease Control and Prevention (CDC) in Atlanta, Georgia, houses about 450 samples; the Russian State Research Center of Virology and Biotechnology near Novosibirsk maintains an inventory of about 120 isolates. Each facility has instituted internationally approved safety standards, backed up by periodic inspections, until the date of final disposition arrives. The CDC inventory, for example, is tightly guarded and stored in the most secure portions of the Atlanta facility, and officials there are reluctant to describe the protections in detail.

With those final test tubes, the story of smallpox concludes—or at least the medical dimension of the story, after some 3,000 years of terror, death, and suffering, is at last drawing to a close.

CHAPTER 2

THE BIOLOGY OF VIRUSES

Viruses are remarkable little creatures. A group of parasitic microscopic organisms that are capable of growth and reproduction only inside the cells of another living thing, they are generally much smaller than other infectious agents, such as bacteria, and are structurally simple, even primitive. There are probably millions of different kinds, perhaps more than all other biological entities or organisms combined, and they exist across the full spectrum of ecological niches: in air, in water, in soil, and inside virtually all living things.

A wide range of highly specialized viruses—of different sizes, shapes, composition, and characteristics—afflicts millions of people, animals, plants, and bacteria annually, with a variety of often incurable diseases. Humans have identified only a small percentage of the multiple genres of viruses, and despite science's long-standing investment in virology, and the rich learning accumulated about viruses, we have only begun to understand how they operate.[1]

The word *virus* is derived from the Latin root for "poison," and various strains of virus are implicated in perhaps 60 percent of the infective diseases around the world. Yet at the same time, many viruses are relatively benign, living without causing damage in their hosts, and some are sought out—it is a contagious mosaic virus that causes the striking variegation in the petals of flowering plants such as Rembrandt tulips, pansies, and gladiolus.

In one sense, a virus is simplicity itself: it has stripped away all nonessential elements and reduced the biological process to its most elemental, parasitic terms. Yet, in other ways, viruses seem highly evolved: each one is specialized for a particular slot in the food chain, and each performs its single function with efficiency.

As a group, viruses are tiny, ranging from ten to four hundred nanometers in diameter. The smallest are barely larger than ribosomes or other internal structures found inside normal cells; the largest (e.g., variola) are almost the size of small bacteria. Some viruses can be detected under a sophisticated light microscope, but for most only an electron microscope will serve. For generations, therefore, even the best scientists were essentially guessing about the structure, nature, and functioning of viruses, entities they could observe only indirectly. The first actual sighting of a variola virus—the first virus of any sort so visualized—came in 1947, under an electron microscope.

Although the structures of different viruses can vary enormously, most share certain characteristics. At the center is a virion, a protective core of protein and a shred of nucleic acid, either DNA or RNA—the virus's genome—formed into one or more strands, loops, or matched pairs. This protein chain may be only five genes long, or it could contain several hundred genes. The simplest viral genome has the blueprint for a handful of proteins; the most complex can elicit hundreds. In the case of the smallpox virus, the genome is a single, relatively lengthy, strip of double-stranded DNA, comprising about two hundred genes. The DNA sequence of different strains of poxviruses are up to 95 percent identical to that of variola; the most critical differences—influencing host-virus interactions and virulence—seem to lie at the ends of the chains.

This viral nucleic acid is surrounded by a protein coat known as a capsid, which protects the virion from the environment, aids in its transportation, and provides a mechanism for inserting it into target cells. Capsid sheaths come in various shapes, such as helical, icosahedral (containing twenty equilateral triangular faces), and spherical. The smallpox virus capsid is often described as ellipsoid or brick shaped. Many viruses, including variola, are often enveloped, with the capsid housed inside an outer membrane made of proteins, carbohydrates, and lipids, which provides, in the case of variola, an overall spherical appearance. The complete variola package, therefore, measures about 250 × 200

× 200 nanometers, making it almost the largest virus. The surface of its outer membrane is studded with irregular tubules.

The infection process begins when a virus approaches a target cell; forcible entry into the cell may then be accomplished in several different ways. Some antibacterial viruses mechanically drill a hole in the cell's outer structure and inject the viral DNA through it, much like the operation of a hypodermic syringe, with the now empty capsid remaining outside. Viruses that afflict plants often enter passively through a microtear in the cell wall. For most animal-affecting viruses, such as variola, the virus waits to be engulfed by the cell membrane, by a process known as endocytosis. In some cases, the virus will affix itself only to specific receptor proteins on a particular cell's outer membrane, and the viral envelope may have discrete glycoprotein (structures that combine carbohydrates with amino acids) spikes that can recognize and bind to the three-dimensional structures that are found only on those designated types of human or animal cells.

In the case of variola, research indicates that the virus seeks out and attaches to host cell receptors that ordinarily bind epidermal growth factor.[2] Entry of the variola virus into the cell occurs in one of two ways, depending on whether the virion is equipped with the usual envelope. If the virus is naked, its outer membrane fuses with the plasma membrane of the target cell and it is engulfed inside a vacuole, drawn inside the cell via a process of invagination, and eventually released into the cell's cytoplasm. If the virus is encased in an envelope, it is absorbed more rapidly and efficiently, spreading the infection with greater speed.[3]

Once the virus has been drawn inside the cell, it sheds the envelope and capsid in two stages, releasing the viral nucleic acid. Although in most other kinds of viruses the DNA then proceeds to penetrate the host cell's nucleus, and destroy or at least suppress the native genetic material there, variola does its damage while remaining entirely within the host's cytoplasm. The virus nonetheless begins to take over the cellular algorithm, hijacking the native machinery with remarkable speed and to a great degree. The variola DNA first inhibits the cell's normal functioning, including self-replication; the cell's energy is devoted, instead, to replication of the virus. Variola is remarkably self-contained for this purpose; it carries with it most of the enzymes needed to accomplish its purposes—most other viruses must commandeer at least some cellular enzymes. New copies of variola DNA are mass-produced, beginning as soon as two to six hours after cellular invasion, and the necessary capsids and envelopes are synthesized, as well—complete new variola particles can be constructed within eight hours.

In effect, the host cell is converted into a miniature variola factory, generating as many copies of the original virus as it can physically hold—about 10,000 to 100,000 viral particles per cell. These copies are emitted through the cell membrane, oozing out in complete, mature, and fully infectious form. Eventually, the cell may burst, releasing thousands of new viruses, each of which can locate, adhere to, and invade other cells. This viral multiplication can proceed at an exponential rate, corrupting millions of cells, damaging tissues and organs, and, ultimately, jeopardizing the organism as a whole.

The defenses that the human body—and modern medicine—erect against many other types of infections are often less effective against viruses. That is, in response to an invasion by a foreign pathogen, a mammal's immune system identifies the specific antigens (the unique marker molecules on the surface of the virus, bacterium, or other threat) and produces appropriate antibodies (proteins that fit the alien envelope's protruding glycoproteins and disrupt the invader by clogging its receptors, gluing multiple invaders together, or directly destroying them).

But viruses pose exceptional challenges to the immune system. Some of these aggressors—the influenza virus is the best example—undergo very frequent mutation, altering the external configuration of those glycoproteins, and thereby fooling or evading the antibodies. In addition, because a virus causes most of its harm while already inside the target cell, many conventional medicines are unable to stop the viral activities without damaging the infected host cells. And in the molecular arms race between the invading virus and the defending host cell, variola has yet another sophisticated ability: it secretes proteins that can bind to, and thereby neutralize, the body's most powerful natural antiviral agent, interferon gamma.

The principal antiviral treatments are therefore precautionary—they involve artificially stimulating the immune system to produce the appropriate antibodies *before* the host is invaded by the virus, so the body is prepared in advance to defend itself. This may be accomplished in several ways, such as by injecting attenuated or killed virus—that is, a serum in which the viral envelope is preserved, with the distinctive glycoproteins intact but in which the viral DNA has been denatured or destroyed, so no cellular invasion can occur.

Smallpox vaccination, however, consists of exposing the body to a slightly *different* virus—vaccinia—which is similar enough to the lethal variola virus to evoke production of appropriate antibodies but mild enough that it rarely causes profound somatic disruptions. The process works so rapidly that vaccination as late as three to four days after exposure to variola—while the smallpox disease is early in the incubation period—can trigger a sufficient immune response to ward off the illness.

Once the appropriate antibodies have been produced, the immune system's memory is engaged, and the body will then be able to re-create more of those specific antibodies quickly, enabling it to ward off exposure to a subsequent infection from the same kind of virus. That is why, for example, one exposure to smallpox confers lifetime immunity. Vaccination via vaccinia, in contrast, provides a lengthy, but nonpermanent, protection against subsequent variola challenge—apparently the body's memory lapses, and its ability to mass-produce the antibodies quickly in that situation is not fully reliable after a decade or so.

IS A VIRUS "ALIVE"?

A virus is nature's ultimate parasite: it is incapable, by itself, of undertaking the usual array of biological functions. It cannot produce or consume energy, move, grow, or reproduce without first invading a living cell and usurping the host's internal mechanisms.

For this reason, many scientists do not consider variola or any other virus to be truly alive, even in the sense that other simple microorganisms, from bacteria to rickettsia (another family of infectious microorganisms) are considered so. Other authorities would, perhaps more generously, consider viruses to be minimal "living organisms," or, according to various circumlocutions, to lie at least "on the threshold of life," "somewhere between complex aggregates of macromolecules and actual living organisms," or "only half alive at best." In any event, customary biological nomenclature does not apply: viruses are not carried in any of the traditional five kingdoms of life, and their species are not typ-

ically accorded the Latinized names routinely attached to all categories of cellular beings.

At the same time, there is surely something about a virus that makes it
different from a conglomeration of inert chemicals. It has at least a kind of life
potential, a dormant biological presence, that is undeniable. Indeed, common
parlance does refer to viruses as being important actors in the world of living
things; they are routinely studied in biology textbooks, rather than in chemistry
courses; we differentiate between live and killed viral vaccinations; and we recognize different species, strains, or families of them.

The recent discovery of categories of even smaller, and even less lifelike,
infective entities has further obscured the question of deriving a meaningful
definition of life. Prions, proteinlike particles devoid of any nucleic acid, have
been implicated in a variety of degenerative brain diseases, such as scrapie in
sheep, mad cow disease, and Creutzfeldt-Jakob disease in humans, although
their precise operational mechanisms are still unknown. Viroids are a cluster of
similar plant-invading creatures, containing a snippet of RNA but none of the
other usual viral accoutrements. Other newfound microscopic entities, intra-
cellular mobile genetic elements of all description, also challenge our ability to
construct reliable, useful demarcations in the netherworld of biology.[4]

Perhaps, therefore, the conventional scientific definition of life is revealed as
being crabbed, arbitrary, or at least inadequate for capturing all the elements
of concern to us in a situation such as this. Whether this vocabulary debate
fairly influences the moral and other judgments about to be made concerning
the future of variola is considered further in chapter 6.

GENETIC ENGINEERING

Developments in genetic engineering have further complicated the debate over
classifying life. In 1973, just as the WHO Intensified Smallpox Eradication Program was approaching its final stages (see chapter 1), and just as the Biological
Weapons Convention was about to be ratified by the United States and other
participants (see chapter 3), the fundamentals of genetic engineering were
being developed—principles that would later complicate both of those medical and legal advances. Today, genetic engineering augurs to alter the most pro-

found aspects of life, promising (or threatening) a reconstitution of the planet's biological and social processes as profound as those changes triggered by the eighteenth-century Industrial Revolution or the twentieth-century popularization of computers.[5]

A detailed account of genetic engineering, of course, lies well beyond the scope of this book, but a layperson's introduction to the field can help establish the basis for a better understanding of smallpox policy choices and risks. In genetic engineering, the first step is the identification and isolation of a gene of interest—the bit of reproductive chemicals that codes the construction of a protein that expresses a particular trait. A complete and accurate map of the entity's genome can help locate each of its individual genes—the map traces the entire molecular sequence of the organism's DNA. (In the case of variola, researchers have now completed the full mapping sequence for ten distinct strains.) The targeted gene is cut out of the DNA structure, by slicing the strand at precise locations, using chemicals known as restriction enzymes.

The next step is to insert the gene fragment into a mechanical or biological vector, used to propagate or transfer it into the organism of interest. One type of biological vector is a plasmid, a circular DNA molecule found in bacteria that can replicate itself independently and lead the cell to perform a variety of important and observable, but usually nonessential, functions. This plasmid circle is also cut, via the same restriction enzyme, and the target gene is inserted into the loop, which is then closed with the aid of another enzyme known as DNA ligase. The newly stitched genetic strand or loop is referred to as recombinant DNA, because it has successfully integrated the new genetically coded information from a distinct species inside the plasmid's prior nucleic acid chain.

Viruses can serve as another common vector—again, the DNA (or RNA) of the virus is sliced, and the gene to be transferred is precisely spliced into it. (For the sake of safety, the virus is also usually attenuated or denatured, so while it will still be able to invade the target cell, and insert its, now modified, DNA, it will not direct the cell to reproduce many more virions or cause significant illness.) Vaccinia has proven to be an especially valuable vector: it is large enough to manipulate easily, and its simple genetic structure facilitates the cutting, insertion, and reclosure sequence.

The plasmid or virus vector is then introduced to members of the target population, such as a culture of bacteria. These host cells will absorb or be invaded by the new genetic material—and, in effect, be at least partially taken over by it. These host bacteria produce generations of genetically exact copies of themselves, including the altered DNA, through their normal multiplication routines—replication via cloning. The bacteria thereby accumulate a significant mass of small, partially new organisms, each containing the artificially engineered gene.

Through this process, scientists can generate amazing juxtapositions. In 1973, the first genetic engineering breakthrough was a mere curiosity: bio-chemists Stanley Cohen and Herbert Boyer succeeded in implanting a fragment of ribosomal RNA from an African clawed toad into the bacterium *Escherichia coli*. They observed in wonderment as the altered bacteria proceeded to gener-ate quantities of toad RNA—the first time that type of foreign intervention had ever been accomplished. But that success is a parlor trick compared to the feats of genetic creativity in the subsequent decades. Three different concepts of genetic engineering deserve mention.

The first, and simplest, involves harnessing the biological energy and fecun-dity of microscopic creatures such as cousins of the ubiquitous laboratory bacterium *E. coli* to produce large quantities of pharmaceutical proteins. Researchers can insert into the bacteria's DNA a gene coding for the produc-tion of human growth hormone (to treat dwarfism), interferon (to battle can-cer), or insulin (to deal with diabetes). Ordinarily, the human body produces only trace amounts of these vital chemicals, and the expense of creating a work-ing stockpile, to aid those who are deficient, is exorbitant. But when the genet-ically engineered bacteria are set to the task, they generate harvestable quanti-ties. The technique can be scaled up to larger animals; for example, pigs and goats can be transgenically modified to produce significant quantities of human protein C, which assists in controlling blood clotting.

A second adaptation of the new power of this science is gene therapy: treat-ments for people suffering from certain hereditary disorders. For example, severe combined immunodeficiency (SCID) in humans is characterized by inadequate production of white blood cells by the bone marrow, resulting in reduced ability to fight off infections. Often, this anomaly is caused by a defec-tive, or missing, single gene, resulting in underproduction of a single, critical protein. In response, doctors add a healthy copy of that gene (from another per-son) to the RNA of a specialized type of modified retrovirus used as a vector. The altered virus is then introduced in vitro to stem cells that have been extracted from the disease sufferer's bone marrow. The usual viral process then operates, with the new, healthy gene becoming interwoven with the original stem cell's chromosomes. When a sufficient number of stem cells have been altered, they are replaced into the person's bone marrow, and there they begin the production of normal disease-fighting white blood cells. Similar gene augmentation processes—sometimes operating by inserting the desired vector and its genetic baggage directly into the person, instead of using a test-tube intermediary stage—are envisioned (and many trials are currently in progress) for combating many deadly and previously intractable human diseases, including cystic fibrosis, cancer, and Parkinson's disease. In treating cystic fibrosis, for instance, a normal gene from another person, carried for this purpose by a common cold virus, is inhaled by nasal spray; inside the lung cells, the new gene would be taken up by the nucleus and begin to order the production of normal mucus.[6]

A third, equally futuristic concept is the genesis of whole new organisms, sharing some of the characteristics of their diverse parentage. To a limited extent, this type of hybridization has been used for centuries: breeding better strains of cattle, corn, and other species through the selection and mating of individuals with the desired traits. But now, working on the biochemical, genetic level, we may be able to orchestrate a new genesis with much greater finesse, speed, and creativity, hatching creatures of such disparate characteristics that they could never have evolved from nature or selective breeding. Bacteria that gobble oil spills, fix nitrogen more rapidly, and help avoid frost damage to plants can now be precisely calibrated. Plants and animals are somewhat harder to engineer than bacteria, but, even so, crops that secrete their own internal insecticides, yield larger or more nutritious fruit, or grow faster and taller with less water and fertilizer, are on the horizon. Larger, more productive "pharm animals," too, can be imagined, as specialized genes from species that cannot mate naturally are brought together in unprecedented ways, in pursuit of greater livestock variety, nutrition, hardiness, and economy.[7] Whole organs, to deal with the demand for transplants into humans, may be grown in pigs that have been genetically modified to match better with humans (to reduce the risk of rejection). Likewise, transgenic mice or other animals may be created with humanlike immune systems, to serve as experimental models for testing new medicines before they are applied to people.

But some of the genetic-engineering possibilities are at least as problematic as they are appealing, and they have inspired an array of doubts and concerns. Some of the antitechnology sentiments echo the expressions, from long ago, of hostility toward the introduction of Montagu's variolation and Jenner's vaccination, as surveyed in chapter 1: they speak to the unnaturalness of the innovative procedures. There are also material concerns about the safety and reliability of gene therapy and about our ability to avoid unforeseen, disastrous side effects. Considerable consumer resistance to genetically modified foodstuffs exists, although experts differ as to how well founded and long lasting that suspicion may be. On the moral or ethical dimension (as surveyed in greater depth in chapter 6) there are questions about the propriety of manipulating the animal (and especially the human) genetic legacy—certainly about the wisdom of playing God by exact steering of an individual's chromosomes. From a legal perspective, there are concerns about patenting or otherwise regulating the secrets of the human genome and about discrimination against individuals found to possess unfavorable genes. And on the military dimension (as explicated in chapter 3), genetically engineered microbes might become tomorrow's biological weapons of choice, used with precision against currently impregnable targets. The same techniques that offer relief from SCID and other crippling genetic impairments also carry the possibility for inventing and unleashing new genres of hostile agents, against which we have no defenses. These designer bugs could, hypothetically, be fused to exhibit specific characteristics, combining the lethality, persistence, and resistance that elude the current arsenals.

GENETIC ALTERATION OF SMALLPOX

As Matthew Meselson has observed, every major technological innovation, from metallurgy to electronics to internal combustion, has been exploited, sooner or later, for military interests as well as for peaceful purposes, and the emerging biotechnologies are unlikely to be any different in that regard.[8] Genetic examination and manipulation of variola and other related orthopox viruses may be a most fitting example. As noted, vaccinia virus has turned out to be a remarkably successful vector for health researchers, serving as the beast of burden for transporting medicinal genes of various sorts into a range of human and other targets. If that virus can be laden with multiple "hitchhikers," could its more deadly cousin, variola, be similarly adapted as a viral cruise missile for precisely conveying selected scraps of DNA into otherwise inaccessible cells? Variola's unique characteristics, and its arcane ability to evade the human immune system defenses, suggest that it might be turned to either good or evil purposes, offering a remarkable medical boon or a military and terrorist bane.

Serendipity—or ill fate—may play an inevitable role too. Just as nerve gas was discovered before World War II by German chemists who were initially seeking only an improved insecticide, Australian researchers in 2001, who were seeking a novel way to control mice, may have inadvertently opened a new door of military/terrorist interest. The modern virologists, attempting to develop a mouse contraceptive vaccine by genetically altering the mouse pox virus, created instead an unusually deadly strain of the virus. If manipulation of the DNA of a milder member of the orthopox virus family can have such an unforeseen effect, what could we anticipate from more concerted efforts?

Thus, we must face the prospect that malevolent forces, too, could seize upon variola in the biotech era. A reengineered version of the virus might be adapted to propound even more powerful smallpox variants or to communicate not merely one loathsome disease but several simultaneously. Already there have been allegations that the former Soviet Union's military researchers succeeded in precisely this sort of inhuman activity, crafting a "chimera" virus that united the worst aspects of smallpox, Ebola, or other potential biological warfare agents.

Accidents must be taken into account, too. Not even the most prestigious, secure, and punctilious facilities can claim total immunity from mishaps, including potentially quite serious errors with some of the most lethal viral and other substances. A microbiologist at the leading U.S. Army biological laboratory recently contracted glanders, a contagious and sometimes fatal bacterial infection previously used as a biological weapon,[9] and a top British research institute was ordered to pay a $65,000 fine for procedures that risked the release of a deadly viral chimera that combined hepatitis C with dengue fever.[10]

RESEARCH INTO VARIOLA VIRUS AND ITS APPLICATIONS

The variola virus has been a subject of great interest for a small cadre of dedicated researchers, but safety, fiscal, and other restrictions have impeded most efforts to dissect and study it. To date, analysts at the Centers for Disease Control and Prevention in Atlanta and at the Vector laboratory in Novosibirsk, Russia, have completed the DNA sequence of nine strains of variola major and one of variola minor, and additional analysis is under way. The complete code for several such strains is now publicly available on the Internet.

That accomplishment, in pursuit of the full range of variability the virus may possess, was initiated in large measure by a committee, established in the years 1998 to 1999 by the Institute of Medicine (IOM) of the National Academy of Sciences, to advise the U.S. government about future scientific needs for live variola virus. The committee, composed of experts in poxviruses, in virology and immunology more generally, and in allied public health fields, was convened at the behest of the Departments of Defense, Energy, and Health and Human Services, and came to exert a major influence on the public debate, both inside the United States and globally. The IOM committee did not reach any formal conclusions about the desirability of retaining or destroying the variola stocks, but it did supply an authoritative analysis of the potential benefits, in several categories of scientific inquiry, of conducting additional research prior to eradication. For example, the committee concluded that additional genomic analysis of variola's DNA sequence and its surface proteins should be conducted before the last remaining samples could rationally be destroyed.

That committee's recommendation, to develop a better understanding of the DNA structure of variola, even if that required delaying any decision about destruction, was based on the observation that there may be important and interesting, but subtle, differences between the several strains of the virus. The approximately 5 percent difference among poxvirus genomes accounts for the remarkable differences in infectivity, lethality, and human impact.[11] Likewise, two strains of variola have been found to be 99.2 percent identical, yet those marginal differences matter in ways we do not yet understand.[12] The first strains of variola that were sequenced had been derived from samples taken from the Indian subcontinent, and other factors, too, suggest that a broader sampling of the available smallpox materials should be undertaken, in the effort to determine which genetic features are responsible for which behavioral characteristics of this virus.

Despite the interest in the work and the breakthroughs that might be realized through studying live smallpox virus, little investigation has been conducted in the United States over the past twenty years. In part, this shortfall is attributable to the dearth of suitable laboratory suites. Work on intact variola can now be conducted only inside facilities designated as meeting standards for biosafety level 4 (BL-4). Such institutions, incorporating redundant separations between the pathogen and people, are expensive to build and maintain, and they can be cumbersome places in which to work. Only two BL-4 facilities in the United States (at the CDC in Atlanta, and at the Army's Fort Detrick in Frederick, Maryland), and perhaps another four elsewhere in the world, would be suitable for variola operations.[13]

Naturally, there is a high demand for space in these premium laboratories and for the time and attention of the researchers. Any smallpox work, therefore, must compete against other worthy applicants—additional variola efforts would displace activity related to AIDS, Ebola, or other viruses that are still active in the environment and, arguably, present more pressing justifications. While there are proposals to construct additional BL-4 facilities in various locations, the costs and potential opposition from neighbors concerned about the introduction of the most noxious pathogens into their communities impede those efforts.

As a partial compromise, some types of smallpox-related work can be conducted at somewhat lower levels of safety. Where researchers can confine their inquiries to working with only a portion of the virus, or if the DNA strand can be partially obstructed or degraded, in a way that mitigates the danger of a smallpox outbreak or other inadvertent disaster, then the lesser standards of BL-3 may be invoked. Much of the structural analysis of variola, including analysis of individual proteins, can be manipulated in this way. Many more facilities can then become suitable for the efforts, but even there the proper procedures require extensive safety measures. And as noted below, in many of the most interesting and important applications, the only plausible focus of the inquiry will be the fully intact, and fully lethal, virus.

Still, there have been significant efforts, or at least proposed efforts, in this field. In 1995, in conjunction with the U.S. government's internal evaluation of then current proposals at the World Health Organization, the Departments of Defense and of Health and Human Services (HHS) had created an advisory board (similar to the 1998–1999 Institute of Medicine investigation) that recommended additional research efforts before the variola stockpiles would be destroyed. Louis W. Sullivan, Secretary of HHS, provided the board's starting point by announcing at an international health meeting that "there is no scientific reason not to destroy the remaining stocks of the wild virus."[14] Still, the advisory board's proposals included suggestions for further research on antiviral drugs, on current and new vaccines, and on the development of improved animal models for evaluating the candidate antivirals and vaccines. Reportedly, the research effort registered some advances—identifying a drug called cidofovir as a possible therapeutic agent, for example—but seems to have raised almost as many questions as it has resolved.

RESEARCH OBJECTIVES

The 1999 Institute of Medicine study provides the most authoritative analysis of what we might learn from further manipulation of those disparate variola samples. At the top of the list is the possibility of deriving improved antiviral agents for use in the event of any future outbreak of smallpox (or, by extension, of other orthopox virus diseases). At present, there is no efficacious potion for combating variola; while some twenty new chemical and biological antiviral agents have received approval from the U.S. Food and Drug Administration in the past decade, and many additional novel compounds, proteins, and concoctions are under investigation, none has yet been proven effective against smallpox.

The process for developing and certifying a new pharmaceutical is long, expensive (it can consume up to twenty years and $500 million, by one accounting),[15] and exacting; even the tiniest change in any aspect of the dozens or hundreds of candidates may have a profound impact upon the drug's potency, safety, and selectivity. No one can predict how long the search for an effective medicine will take—the analogy to the still fruitless quest for solutions to the problems of influenza and AIDS makes one skeptical that the antivariola research campaign could promise quick success. Moreover, few experts would suggest that private enterprise, unaided by public financial support, would be sufficient to carry the day.

Another significant research application for the variola samples would be to assist in developing an improved vaccine. The previous and existing anti-smallpox vaccines (based on cowpox in Jenner's era, and on vaccinia virus more recently) have over the decades provided heroic service to humanity, but they have important defects. The first problem is availability: the world has maintained a stockpile of 60 to 90 million doses of vaccinia (as much as 6 to 15 million in the United States), but the entire stockpile is aging, and much of it has been stored in suboptimal conditions that jeopardize its continued potency.[16] While a small quantity of seed stocks has also been retained by the WHO, there was little, if any, recent manufacturing of vaccine. The September 11, 2001, terrorist attacks on the World Trade Center and the Pentagon provided the stimulus for a massive new production of vaccine, and the pharmaceutical industry's surge capability for quickly producing more vaccine, in response to the sudden emergency, is sure to be tested by this demand.

Moreover, the vaccinia vaccine—based on a live virus, with infective, albeit, usually mild, properties—carries a long list of side effects and contraindications, especially problematic in an era in which the proliferation of HIV has compromised the immune systems of millions of people. Some have conjectured that the vaccinia vaccine, for all its success, would not be authorized for use by the U.S. Food and Drug Administration today. Even in response to the burgeoning threat of biological terrorism following September 11, 2001, health officials have not decided to resume automatic smallpox vaccination of the general population and have not even determined whether to make the vaccination available on a voluntary basis to those who seek it—perhaps holding the vaccine in a secure national repository, against possible use in an emergency, would still be the safest course. In any event, the hope for improved prophylaxis, built on twenty-first-century medical technology, appears to be a challenging, but realistic and necessary, objective.

A third potential benefit of additional variola research highlighted by the IOM study would be acquisition of more generally applicable insights into virology and human immunology, with potential transference to the struggles against other pathogens. Variola is, after all, an unusual case study, presenting some exceptional characteristics: the virus has repeatedly demonstrated a unique ability to evade human control, insidiously dodging the best efforts of both our natural systems and our artificially constructed pharmaceuticals. It is also a relatively well-studied exemplar, one that humans have engaged in long-standing, minutely documented mortal combat. Further basic and applied investigations, therefore, may be unusually promising, helping to arm our species for future battles against this and other invaders. Especially when we cannot possibly predict the machinations of future technology, how can we be certain that there are no lessons from variola worth pursuing?

Finally, the IOM report outlines two areas of viral detection that call for improvement. First, we might enhance our ability to detect the smallpox virus inside the human body earlier, to confirm a diagnosis and begin appropriate isolation and medical treatment. And we might also accelerate our ability to detect and quickly defend against a virus in the environment, such as an oncoming aerosol cloud of biological weaponry that had been released by a hostile military or terrorist force. Both of those unmet challenges are potentially important, and our abilities in each area have been dormant for decades.

At the same time, there are obstacles that any conscientious research and development program on variola would have to confront. The first, as usual, is money: who will pay for this ambitious set of inquiries? By one estimate, development of a new antiviral drug to combat variola effectively may cost as much as $300 million.[17] Because smallpox as a disease has long been eradicated, there may be no appreciable commercial market for an improved vaccine or new antiviral medicines to combat it. Unless public funds are directed into this field, the private laboratories will surely pursue other, more remunerative, options. For its part, the World Health Organization has no significant funding to devote to such an enterprise. Skeptics could surely question how resolute the U.S. Congress and the executive branch will be in their commitment to provide adequate funding for further research into a dead disease, at a time when other claimants for the limited pot of public funding can press seemingly more urgent claims. Once the current crisis has passed, will smallpox still command the dollars that our fears about bioterrorism have recently inspired?

Second, the fact that variola afflicts only humans—a reality essential to the success of the WHO eradication campaign—complicates any meaningful research protocol. In order to fully study the virus in its natural state, and thereby to gain the most realistic understanding of its functioning and to have confidence in any candidate vaccines or antiviral preparations, we would have to infect human beings with smallpox—a proposal that is patently unacceptable under modern ethical standards. There is, to be sure, a great deal that can be accomplished short of that final step: researchers can manipulate portions of the variola genome or the empty viral envelope; they can experiment with other orthopox viruses in animals, to deduce whether analogous treatments prove efficacious; and they can even construct, via the most sophisticated genetic engineering, transgenic animals (such as mice) that are artificially endowed with a human immune system. Still, lingering doubts will remain about any product or technique that might be developed exclusively through these second-best alternatives; lacking firsthand observation of clinical trials in humans, the U.S. Food and Drug Administration (and its counterpart institutions in other countries, such as the European Medicines Evaluation Agency) would have to adapt their normal protocols and standards in order to endorse any new antivariola products, as the FDA has now started to do.

Finally, it should be noted that research on something less than the intact variola particle can continue, in relative safety and (since something less than BL-4 facilities would be required) at lower cost. Even if the WHO does order the destruction of all variola stocks, and even if the two repository countries comply, researchers might still be allowed to continue work on related, noninfective fragments—for example, DNA plasmids or viral envelopes. For some purposes, that constrained research program could be sufficient. For example, the effort to develop improved field detection and diagnostic routines would not necessarily require access to live variola virus. For other important enterprises, however, the IOM study confirms that some manipulation of the intact, viable virus would be required in order to validate the findings. For example, any new antismallpox vaccine, even after thorough testing with plasmids or other simulants, would still require confirmation via exposure to intact variola.

In November 2001, the Bush administration announced that the United States had determined not to proceed with eradication of the viral samples until researchers were able to satisfy a series of stiff conditions. First, a new vaccine, licensed as safe for the entire community (i.e., not causing the same sorts of adverse side effects as the current vaccine in various health-compromised individuals) must be produced. Second, not one, but two antiviral medications, operating against variola through distinct biological mechanisms, must be generated. (Cidofovir is the most advanced preparation at the moment, but any other candidates were far in arrears.) Third, more reliable diagnostic tests and environmental detectors must be invented. Finally, an ability to defeat genetically altered versions of variola must emerge. Acknowledged as setting the bar for variola destruction quite high—perhaps requiring a decade of additional research—these new criteria quickly met the approval of the senior laboratory official in custody of the Russian variola stocks, but, as described in chapter 5, may encounter resistance from WHO and other member countries.

SOURCES FOR POSSIBLE RENEWAL OF SMALLPOX

Recognition of human fallibility cautions that even if the world succeeds in destroying both the American and Russian repositories of variola, there may still be no guarantee against the virus somehow resurfacing, and the disease reemerging.

Some scenarios for a resurgence of smallpox have already been noted. Security experts in the United States and elsewhere fear that secret variola stockpiles, never declared to the WHO and never surrendered to international authorities, may still exist, buried in military freezers in North Korea, Russia, or elsewhere. As Ken Bernard, the Clinton Administration's top official on the smallpox eradication issue for the National Security Council staff, put it, "We are relatively sure that most of the virus is in the two declared stocks. There's just no way to ensure that if we destroy the two declared stocks that we will destroy every smallpox virus that exists."[18] Hostile forces—covertly controlled by unrepentant national authorities or by rogue elements that operate independently of effective centralized governmental direction—may have stashed variola stocks, despite their country's overt acceptance of the Biological Weapons Convention and despite any WHO action.

It is also possible that other laboratories may continue to house variola repositories more by accident than by design: within a large laboratory, hospital, or research freezer might be samples of smallpox residues, poorly labeled, inadequately inventoried, and long forgotten—but still viable. After all, not long ago smallpox was still a global disease, with infectious materials present everywhere, for legitimate diagnostic, analytical, research, and other purposes. As smallpox expert D. A. Henderson puts it, "Virologists are like squirrels. A lot of this stuff goes in deep freezes . . . at no time could you ever say, no matter what you did, that there was no smallpox [virus] anywhere."[19] Errant variola residues have been discovered before, in California in 1979, in Tanzania in 1979, and perhaps in London in 1985.[20]

Today's standards for materials accountancy should minimize the dangers, but even the best facilities may continue to be the subject of plausible rumors about covert variola stocks, and it can be difficult, tiresome, and expensive to prove the negative, as the U.S. National Institutes of Health recently discovered. An anonymous 1995 allegation that the highly respected Bethesda, Maryland, laboratory housed secret variola stocks resulted in a lengthy exploration of thousands of frozen samples and their accompanying documentation, without finding anything untoward.

In addition to those low-technology dangers, three other scenarios building more upon the biotechnology revolution are worth considering.

The first possibility is almost a nonfiction reprise of Michael Crichton's 1991 thriller *Jurassic Park* and the spectacular effort by misguided scientists to revive the dinosaurs by building from microscopic remnants of their DNA preserved in prehistoric amber. Here, the scenario is that viable variola particles may be contained in the corpses of people felled by smallpox long ago, especially those who lived and died suddenly in frigid northern climates, where the bodies were buried in the permafrost, lost in Ice Age caves, or encased by glaciers where they happened to fall. The thought is that the virus might remain intact for decades, or even centuries, in those sterile, dry, cold conditions, subject to being revived if the tomb were carefully warmed.

We know little about the sustainability of variola or other viruses in those cryogenic conditions: there are widely divergent estimates about the viability of variola even at room temperatures, and there has been no experience with recovery of infective particles after many years, let alone centuries, of isolation. We do know, however, that active genetic material has recently been extracted from influenza virus particles drawn from eighty-year-old laboratory tissue samples preserved from deceased 1918 Spanish flu victims.[21] And some especially hardy viruses and other microbes—the anthrax bacillus, another potential biological warfare agent, comes readily to mind—can persist in inert spores in the environment for long periods.

Scientists who may potentially encounter such long-dormant viral residues are concerned, and a modest debate has ensued in the literature about whether there is any danger to paleontologists who come into contact with the corpses of smallpox-infested cave dwellers. Likewise, those who traverse formerly variola-infested areas (e.g., abandoned smallpox hospitals or cemeteries) worry about their potential exposure if excavation or modern economic development were to churn up dust and long-dormant germs. Russian researchers have occasionally attempted to seek out and exhume the frozen remains of possible smallpox victims to determine the plausibility of this novel theory; to date their results have been inconclusive.

A different scenario involves an outbreak in humans of monkey pox, an evolving, potentially quite lethal viral cousin of smallpox. A member of the diverse orthopox virus family, monkey pox is not a new disease, having been observed in primates and squirrels since at least 1958, and in people since 1970, but it seems to have experienced increased incidence in humans, especially in its transmissibility from one person to another.

Monkey pox has historically been observed principally in remote villages of Central and West Africa, in and around the tropical rain forests where humans have the most frequent contact with infected animals. The disease is most commonly spread to people through contamination from an animal's blood or a bite. Once thought to be a disappearing problem, monkey pox has made a strong return, due to some combination of mutation in its viral genome and behavioral changes in nearby human population groups. For example, in recent years, ongoing civil war in the Democratic Republic of the Congo (DROC, formerly Zaire) has provided the backdrop for a noticeable increase in human monkey pox occurrences there, perhaps prompted by war refugees seeking shelter in increasingly remote jungles and turning to monkey meat as a source of food.

In the past, the occasional eruption of a monkey pox infection was isolated and short-lived, because it was not routinely passed from one person to the next, and it rarely succeeded in spreading beyond that second generation. Therefore, despite the fact that the disease carried a fatality rate of 10 percent (and was highest among children) it gained little notoriety.[22] Recently, however, the situation has deteriorated. Some 511 suspected monkey pox cases were reported in the DROC in 1996 to 1997 and fully 78 percent of those suspect cases had been passed from one person to the next, instead of being acquired directly from an animal source.[23]

The World Health Organization and many others are concerned that a slightly mutated monkey pox virus may now pose a substantial public health problem in Africa and potentially beyond. If the virus has somehow evolved into a form that facilitates its transfer between people, then a crisis may be looming. The monkey pox virus is similar (both genetically and in its effects) to variola, and the cross-immunity is strong (anyone who has been exposed to either—or to vaccinia—is generally immune to the other). There have been proposals to reintroduce a widespread vaccinia vaccination program into the West African rain forest, despite the aforementioned problems with both the quantity and safety of the existing vaccine.

The fact that the monkey pox virus, unlike variola, is sustained in animals makes it even more problematic—it cannot be eradicated simply by protecting exposed people, because the virus could readily retreat to its jungle reservoir, being passed from monkey to monkey indefinitely, until a vulnerable person becomes exposed and reinitiates a chain or epidemic. As Peter Jahrling, a leading U.S. Army virologist, puts it, "I hate to be accused of pushing the alarmist button, but for practical purposes, smallpox is back."[24]

Finally, there is the no longer simply futuristic scenario of reconstituting variola. We have a complete DNA map of the virus, and we have an increasing ability to stitch nucleotide chains together chemical by chemical; might it be possible for researchers to reassemble the variola genome "from scratch," even if all known exemplars, fragments, and infectious residues were permanently destroyed?

The finesse and knowledge necessary to create viral life artificially are now within reach, and a primitive example has already been accomplished, for research purposes, with the Ebola virus and more recently with the polio virus. If the technique can be perfected, with the resulting molecule acquiring the spark of whatever it is that allows a virus to perform its customary viral functions, then a new era of playing God will have arrived.

Variola may be a propitious target for that sort of bioengineering. It has long been observed that those poxviruses that infect vertebrates exhibit a unique property of natural nongenetic reactivation or transfection; that is, if a target cell is simultaneously infected with both a killed, but physically intact, variola virion and a live copy of some other member of the orthopox family, the enzymes from the latter can help reconstitute and unleash the former, and fully communicable smallpox is produced. Moreover, there is no technical impediment to the eventual establishment of a laboratory capability for creating infectious poxviruses from synthetic DNA fragments. As the Institute of Medicine committee observed, "It is entirely possible that future advances in gene synthesis and transfection technologies would enable synthesis of variola virus from the published sequence information." The committee added, "There is no way of predicting the rate at which such technologies might develop."[25]

In fact, the genetic engineers would not have to begin their construction of a variola particle truly from scratch. They might, instead, use more sophisticated starting points, such as the virion from some other member of the orthopox virus family, or even noninfectious portions of the variola DNA that might legitimately be preserved after the main laboratory samples had been incinerated. If that type of manipulation can be accomplished, it suggests the futility of ordering the destruction of all current variola stockpiles.

THE PRECEDENT FOR THE NEXT ERADICATED VIRUS

The world has never before managed to subdue and confine an entire species of virus, in the way it has done with variola. Other notorious pathogens still remain at large, with at least sporadic (or much larger, persistent, and deadly) outbreaks and with human efforts, led by the World Health Organization or others, to defeat the diseases still struggling. The glorious 1967 to 1979 global smallpox enterprise, therefore, not only stands as an inspiration to those who would sponsor a similar effort to rid the world of other infectious scourges, it also serves to warn that the effort may turn out to be far more expensive, difficult, and uncertain than its advocates might initially imagine.

Moreover, many of these viruses and other microscopic organisms, the erstwhile candidates for an intensified eradication campaign, seem fated to elude human enterprise and conquest indefinitely. Some are sufficiently nonselective or adaptable to hide inside the biological systems of wild animals or elsewhere, even if nonimmune human hosts were to become temporarily unavailable. Some do not manifest themselves right away in an obvious, debilitating form, so an asymptomatic carrier could unwittingly transmit them over a wide area. Some have not yet yielded to an effective vaccine, and even the most earnest researchers do not promise that a safe, effective, and affordable preventative measure is on the horizon.

In fact, new viral threats seem to emerge with frightening regularity these days. Within the past decades, HIV has spread around the world, hemorrhagic fevers such as hantavirus and Ebola have been identified, and, most recently, West Nile virus has traveled from Africa into the United States. Other infectious diseases have adapted to enter the human system from domestic or feral animal sources. We seem to be suffering from "an epidemic of epidemics," as Anne Platt McGinn puts it,[26] and most of these emerging threats are still without preventative cure or treatment.

Still, some notorious diseases have yielded to human technology and persistence, and a few have emerged as plausible candidates for foreseeable eradication. The virus causing poliomyelitis, for example, had long been considered extinct in the Americas—until a reemergence of four paralyzing cases in the Dominican Republic and Haiti in 2000. Like variola, polio has no animal reservoir to retreat to, and, also like variola, the disease it causes has elicited a concerted, and now reasonably well-funded, global campaign to defeat it.

In recent years, a vigorous outreach campaign has immunized vast numbers of people, especially young children: 134 million people were vaccinated in India in a single day in 1997, and organizers planned to exhaust some 2.5 billion doses in 2000. Correspondingly, the number of new polio cases has plummeted, from 350,000 in 1988 to perhaps 7,000 in 1999 and as few as 600 in 2001.[27] New money, human energy, and a high-profile global effort, marked by an unusually cooperative spirit—including even suspension of wars in order to allow mass vaccination to proceed—have begun to pay off.

The world seems close to total victory over the polio virus (which is different from variola in size, configuration, and perhaps in infective processes). While much work remains to be done (the disease is still endemic in fifty countries) and the original target dates for completion may slip again, by the end of 2005 polio may be virtually eradicated. After a suitable two- to five-year period of uneventful observation, the WHO would be able to certify the global triumph over a second deadly disease.

Quite likely, therefore, the polio virus will be the next microbe to be confined to isolation in laboratory freezers—and perhaps the next in line for consideration for total extermination of its species. Some WHO officials have already anticipated those eventualities, proposing guidelines for locating the world's polio virus holdings, consolidating them, and upgrading their security. Scores of laboratories and other facilities in many countries still hold infectious polio materials of various sorts, perhaps without even recognizing them as such, and WHO is anxious to avoid repetition of the smallpox laboratory accidents in London and Birmingham, England, in 1973 and 1978.

After that, global health officials may turn their attention to eradication of a variety of nonviral diseases. Dracunculiasis, or "guinea worm fever," is a debilitating disease caused by a parasitic worm and is spread by contaminated drinking water. It infected some 3.6 million people in 1986, but modern water purification and filtration techniques have reduced it to fewer than 90,000 cases in 1999, all in sub-Saharan Africa.[28] Likewise, a twenty-year public health campaign has made progress in conquering parasitic onchocerciasis, or "river blindness," and improved vaccines have just about stopped the African cattle virus disease rinderpest.

Other noxious microbes, however, seem even more resistant. The measles virus, for example, while mostly a relatively minor, and now rare, childhood inconvenience in the United States, is still a major killer elsewhere, with deaths reaching one million annually. The disease has motivated a global vaccination campaign, and the WHO has targeted 2013 as the date for eradication. Yet, the current vaccine is imperfect in its protection and durability, and in some communities the relatively trivial nature of the disease has resulted in low rates of vaccination of susceptible individuals.

Likewise, the virus that causes yellow fever, the bacterium that causes bubonic plague, and the parasite that causes malaria have shown stubborn resistance to eradication attempts. While dedicated efforts have resulted in saving millions of lives, few would claim that the last vestiges of these causative agents will soon follow variola into a test-tube confinement. Some, such as the bacterium that causes tuberculosis, seem to be evolving in a worse direction: multidrug-resistant tuberculosis is now a major new threat, reviving fears that humanity had once thought were largely put to rest.

The crystal ball thus becomes dim as we try to look more than just a few years into the future of microbiology, and it becomes completely opaque as we try to discern precisely which microbes will be placed on humanity's chopping block, in what order, and on what timetable. Still, the big picture emerges: the biological, ethical, legal, and other considerations that we are now wrestling with in the context of smallpox and variola are not unique; they will be repeated, fairly frequently, perhaps in slightly different form and in somewhat different context, for other illnesses and pathogens, and probably sooner rather than later.

CONCLUSION

Modern microbiology brings us both unprecedented power and unprecedented danger. The technology offers us the promise of conquering disease; a fair regard for humility, of course, suggests that we should not predict that we will be able to cure all diseases or solve any of the major pathogenic riddles very soon, but the human curiosity and resourcefulness in this area are inexorable. As we learn more about viral operations and their infective pathways, surely our understanding will yield additional tools to supplement the body's natural defenses in resounding ways.

What is less clear is whether we will have the wisdom to wield this newfound prowess with grace and discretion. Cellular operations demand a supreme delicacy, a technique that is now within reach; but they should surely also demand a certain deftness of judgment that our species has not always exhibited. The adaptability of genetic engineering techniques to hostile weapons purposes, for example, demonstrates that there is no innovation so inspired, no human accomplishment so magnificent, that it cannot be distorted to evil ends. Just as we celebrate the human enterprise that enabled the conquest of smallpox and has brought us to the brink of success against polio and other afflictions, we must confront the prospect that artificial manipulation of the viral genome might produce chimerical creatures combining the worst aspects of multiple deadly diseases.

The primary lessons of this inquiry, therefore, are that the biotechnology revolution is already in full swing; that its powers are more immense, and its dangers more pronounced, than the general public may appreciate; and that there seems to be little we can do to direct, impede, or channel it. This is not essentially future technology to ponder; it is current technology, already being applied in breathtaking fashion.

The biological dimension of the variola eradication story, therefore, contributes insights into both human strength and human limitations. There is still much more that could be learned from further examination of this virus; whether we have the money, time, facilities, patience, incentive, and will to do so—and whether we possess the self-restraint to do so exclusively for benign purposes—remains to be seen.

CHAPTER 3

smaLLpox as a BIoLogical weapon

Biological weaponry (BW) has never been at the forefront of any army's arsenal. There are too many other more accessible, equally deadly, and less despicable alternatives competing for attention and funding. Moreover, most traditional biological weapons have suffered important, well-known weaknesses or practical limitations that undercut their potential battlefield utility.[1]

Nevertheless, the weaponeers in many countries have long persisted in their biological inquiries, and an extraordinary creativity has been marshaled through the centuries in the attempt to turn to military purposes the fundamental lessons of the life sciences. Today, the biotechnology revolution threatens to accelerate that process, turning the anti-BW consensus on its head, as new iterations of germ weaponry may become more manageable, lethal, and selective than their primitive natural predecessors could ever have been.

The history of biological weaponry is inextricably linked to the history of chemical weaponry (CW)—only in this century has our vocabulary even attempted a precise demarcation between those categories. Essentially, a biological weapon (such as smallpox or anthrax) is one relying on a living organism (or on infective material derived from such an agent) that causes a (lethal or other) disease by reproducing itself inside humans, animals, or plants. A chemical weapon (such as mustard gas or nerve gas), in partial contrast, relies upon a substance—in solid, liquid, or gaseous form—that causes direct toxic effects (deadly or incapacitating, long or short term) to the tissues, organs, or bodily functioning. A "toxin weapon" (such as rattlesnake poison or tricothecene) occupies a sort of middle ground: it consists of chemical substances produced naturally by living organisms (and, with inevitable confusion, also the various synthetically produced analogues of those natural substances) that can directly harm a target, without reproducing themselves inside it or creating a "disease." These protodefinitions are at best approximations for categories that no longer admit precise splicing—but the acknowledgment that we inevitably are dealing with something of a gray area may be the best we can do.

EVOLUTION OF CHEM-BIO WARFARE

Accounts of ancient experimentation with what we would now term chemical and biological weaponry are interpreted today as a polyglot mixture of mythology, propaganda, psychological combat, and perhaps even a small quantity of true military effectiveness. Classical Indian (1500–500 B.C.), Greek (400 B.C.), and Roman (100 B.C.) literature each abounds with lurid depictions of the application of various types of poisons as enhancements of an attacker's offensive weaponry (what military lingo now designates as a "force multiplier"). Typically, these involved the creation of "poison arrows" or other extraordinary projectiles, or the dispatching of covert agents to insert devastating additives into an enemy's water sources and food supplies.

Solon of Athens, for example, is reported to have used the noxious roots of the helleborus plant—a primitive but effective toxin weapon—to poison the water supply of the city of Kirra in 600 B.C., and Alexander the Great, among others, may have catapulted infected corpses into besieged cities. Some have even speculated that the fifth of the ten plagues visited by Moses upon ancient Egypt, referred to as "morrain," may have been the disease we now know as anthrax. Whether any of these ancient tactics had any true impact upon their targets is debatable, but the concept of exploiting biology and chemistry for hostile purposes was certainly well-established long before New Testament times.

The succeeding centuries witnessed piecemeal invocations of that strategy, with armies occasionally deliberately using diseased human or animal corpses to foul each other's rivers and wells in the effort to spread debilitating illness. Early military strategists recognized that incapacitating an enemy soldier might sometimes be more advantageous than killing him—a sick or injured belligerent consumed far more of his colleagues' time, energy, and resources than did a dead one. But the medical technology of the earlier eras was so underdeveloped, and the social understanding of disease processes was so primitive, that even the most pernicious generals were unable to exploit this potential as fully as they might have wished.

At the same time, however, *accidental* use of "biological weapons agents" was ubiquitous and singularly momentous. In virtually every war, far more people—soldiers and civilians alike—have been debilitated and killed by disease than by any combination of arrows, bullets, and bombs.[2] The stresses of wartime—usually accompanied by a scarcity of nourishment and fuel, prolonged exposure to the harsh elements, and living in close quarters—provide an ideal breeding ground for communicable illnesses. Far surpassing any military commander's ability to plan and control, disease outbreaks have changed the course of history, altering the outcomes of battles and triggering the rise and fall of empires.

Public opinion, too, has played a major role in the evolution of biochemical warfare. People everywhere have recoiled against the incorporeal forms of combat, regarding them as sneaky, dishonorable, illegitimate, or unfair—even while their own forces were still contemplating, preparing for use, or even using the identical potions and poisons. The same ancient civilizations that recorded incidents of the occasional adoption of toxic weapons simultaneously hand down to us a precursor international law or ethic purporting to restrict or abolish them. The Indian *Atharva Veda* and the cognate Greek and Roman military codes, for example, express an abhorrence of these "unconventional" weapons, even while those proscriptions were frequently honored only in the breach.

Through the Middle Ages, both the episodic military use of poison weapons and public and legal disdain for them accelerated. A now infamous fourteenth-century incident (often cited as the first confirmed application of a biological weapon in combat) highlighted both the military attraction and the public loathing of BW. There, Janibeg, khan of a Kipchak Tartar army besieging the Crimean city of Kaffa (now known as Feodosiia, Ukraine), catapulted plague-infested cadavers over the city walls in the effort to trigger an epidemic among the defenders of the city of 50,000 inhabitants. Genoan merchants, subsequently fleeing the city, then managed to transport the plague throughout the known world by 1347 to 1348, with devastating consequences for the population of Europe. Still, it is not clear that it was the alien corpses that had truly initiated the city's—and then the world's—most monumental illness.

Condemnation of such practices by the international legal authorities of the day was unequivocal (if not always completely effectual). Alberico Gentili declared in 1598 that "it is a guileful deed when we desire to make use of poison, and one which is not admitted even against the enemy." He articulated a family of no fewer than nineteen reasons why poisons should not be employed on the battlefield, including the assertions that it was done by barbarians, that it was too cruel, that it was "a violation of nature," and that it was "contrary to the laws of the Gods and the manners of our forefathers."[3]

Hugo Grotius, widely acknowledged as "the father of international law," asserted in 1625 that "from old times the law of nations—if not of all nations, certainly those of the better sort—has been that it is not permissible to kill an enemy by poison."[4] Likewise, Emmerich de Vattel argued, "The use of poisoned weapons is nevertheless prohibited by the law of nature, which does not allow us to multiply the evils of war beyond all bounds. . . . Besides, if you poison your weapons, the enemy will follow your example; and thus, without gaining any advantage . . . you have only added to the cruelty and calamities of war."[5]

Still, the concept remained in the public and the military consciousness: Shakespeare's works contain no fewer than 123 references to poison, and even Leonardo da Vinci at least briefly turned his genius to the task of designing a novel device for more effectively dispensing lethal substances in combat.

Smallpox has played a conspicuous role in this convoluted military history. As noted in chapter 1, the ambitions of ancient empires from the Egyptians to the Hittites to the Athenians alternately benefited and suffered from the caprice of the variola virus. Accidental smallpox epidemics—spread unknowingly, but with awesome effectiveness, by Spanish conquistadores—devastated the Aztec, Mayan, and Inca civilizations of Central and South America. Likewise, the eighteenth-century French and British efforts for control of North America were sporadically aided and constrained by ongoing struggles with the disease.

Even deliberate use of a smallpox weapon was not out of the question. In

1763, during "Pontiac's Rebellion," at the latter stages of the French and Indian War, Sir Jeffrey Amherst, Britain's North American commander-in-chief (who was well acquainted, from long experience, with the devastating effects of disease on military order and operational effectiveness), proposed biological warfare. In a July 7 letter to his subordinate, Colonel Henry Bouquet, the ranking officer for western Pennsylvania, Amherst suggested, "Could it not be Contrived to Send the *Small Pox* among those Disaffected Tribes of Indians? We must, on this occasion, Use Every Stratagem in our power to Reduce them."[6]

Bouquet wrote back to Amherst on July 13: "I will try to inoculate the ____ with Some Blankets that may fall in their Hands, and take care not to get the disease myself."[7] Amherst, apparently satisfied, responded shortly thereafter, "You will Do well to try to Inoculate the Indians, by means of Blankets, as well as to Try Every other Methode, that can Serve to Extirpate this Execrable Race." Shortly thereafter, defenders of Fort Pitt (near what is now the city of Pittsburgh), led by British Captain Simeon Ecuyer, conspired to pass, ostensibly as a token of friendship, two blankets and one handkerchief delicately removed from a local smallpox hospital to two hostile chiefs, in the hope that "it will have the desired effect."[8]

While the historical record remains obscure about whether the scheme was consummated, by the following spring, smallpox was indeed raging among the unsuspecting "savage" Indians in the Ohio River valley, and sixty to eighty Mingoes, Delawares, and Shawanoes had died of an infection resembling smallpox. Still, it is not certain whether the contemplated British intervention had been its trigger; there were many other possible sources for the outbreak at that time.

Historians have concluded that there were numerous incidents in which French, Spanish, and English colonizers used or threatened to use smallpox, whether deliberately, accidentally, or merely taking advantage of natural outbreaks among the Native Americans "as an ignoble means to an end."[9] And there may have been some comparable efforts in reverse—attempts by the Iroquois and Cree tribes to use smallpox or other diseases as weapons against the whites or against each other.

A crude version of what we might now deem an individual terrorist's use of a smallpox weapon may have had some eighteenth-century precedent. According to some reports, a white trader, furious at the loss of some of his equipment to Indian raiders, exacted his revenge by perfidiously inviting their tribal leaders to smoke a peace pipe and then presenting them with a keg of rum wrapped in a blanket that had been contaminated with the variola virus. When they carried the Trojan horse gift back to their village, it triggered a smallpox outbreak that proved fatal for many.

There were likewise unproven, but highly suggestive, allegations of the deliberate use of smallpox as a weapon in the succeeding one hundred years, including during the American Revolutionary War. Defending against intense sieges of Boston and later of Quebec City, British forces sent recently inoculated civilians outside the city fortifications to mingle with unprotected Continental Army troops, hoping to spread smallpox among them and fatally weaken the attacks.[10]

During the American Civil War, diseases of all sorts taxed military officials on both sides, impeding their training, maneuvers, and military operations. Most of this illness (including the incidence of smallpox) was undoubtedly natural in origin, but there were persistent reports of the intentional spreading of smallpox and perhaps of crude efforts at biological terrorism involving deliberate introduction of yellow fever into Northern cities. Certainly, the commanders attempted to exploit each other's exposure to variola (e.g., trying to pin enemy forces in locations where the disease was known to be raging), and neither side was able to take great comfort in vaccination, which remained an inexact art.

Through the nineteenth century, states and academic commentators continued to rail against chemical and biological weaponry, although the vocabulary for making that distinction had not yet emerged, and although—more important—proposals continued for military applications of poisons. During the American Civil War, the Lieber Code, promulgated as a Union General Order in 1863, led the way by declaring "The use of poison in any manner, be it to poison wells, or food, or arms, is wholly excluded from modern warfare. He that uses it puts himself out of the pale of law and usages of war."[11] Upon its heels, the 1868 Declaration of St. Petersburg, the 1874 Declaration of Brussels, and the Hague Conferences in 1899 and 1907 invoked the horror of poison weapons and deepened the international community's expression of outrage against them—just as that consensus was about to be shattered by the conduct manifested by all sides during World War I.

TWENTIETH-CENTURY
ARMAMENTS AND ARMS CONTROL

From the German trenches near Ypres, Belgium, on April 22, 1915, emerged the first sustained applications of modern lethal chemical weaponry, terrifying the unprepared victims. A wave of dense yellow smoke (later identified as chlorine gas released by the Kaiser's forces from 5,730 emplaced cylinders) asphyxiated two panicked French divisions and instantly gutted the long-standing international taboo against toxic arms. Thereafter, clouds of mustard gas, phosgene, cyanide, and other hazards (a total of 130,000 tons of fifty-four separate substances) regularly floated back and forth along the ragged European front— largely without telling military advantage to either side—for the duration of the Great War. The bestiary of gases accounted for perhaps 1.25 million military casualties, of whom approximately 100,000 died.[12]

The Kaiser's forces also found a way to use biological weapons against the Allies' cattle, cavalry, and draft animals, if not their troops. German spies and saboteurs were apprehended in the United States, Russia, Romania, Argentina, and elsewhere, attempting to infect cattle with anthrax and horses and mules with glanders (another highly infectious animal disease). By systematically contaminating livestock and animal feed even in neutral countries that shipped such goods to the allies, Germany apparently hoped to undermine its opponents' war efforts.

After the armistice, the world renewed its struggle to proscribe future poison wars, which the public resoundingly considered illegitimate. The Treaty of Versailles tried to drive the noxious genie back into its bottle by explicitly prohibiting Germany from rearming itself with toxic weapons, and in an uncommon act of self-denial the victorious United States, United Kingdom, France, Italy, and Japan each shortly thereafter pledged to itself reject the implements of chemical warfare. The key development, however, came with the negotiation of the Geneva Protocol, signed by twenty-nine countries on June 17, 1925.

This treaty—incredibly brief, when compared to the excruciating length and detail of modern arms control documents—bars "the use in war of asphyxiating, poisonous or other gases, and of all analogous liquids, materials or devices." At the urging of the prescient Polish representative, the parties further agreed "to extend this prohibition to the use of bacteriological methods of warfare."[13] The Geneva Protocol attracted some forty-three parties during the interwar period (the United States and Japan stood out as prominent holdouts until the 1970s)—at the time, a significant percentage of the world's leading powers. Simultaneously, the notion grew that use of chemical or biological weapons—or at least the first, offensive use—should be appreciated as a violation of "customary international law," binding upon all countries irrespective of their membership in, or absence from, any specific treaty regime embodying some version of the overarching principle.

But the Geneva Protocol suffered important shortcomings. For starters, it constituted merely a nonuse commitment; there was no restriction on the development, production, and deployment of the regulated arms. In addition, through a series of "reservations" submitted by many states, they each retained the right to employ chemical or biological weapons generally against any nonparty state, and even against a party to the protocol, if that party were guilty of using those weapons first—effectively converting the accord into a partial, no *first* use pledge. Third, the treaty also contained no inspection procedures or other mechanisms for verifying compliance; nor did it offer any institutional "enforcement" structure for dealing responsibly with disputes or violations.

Finally, of greatest relevance here, the negotiators' limited understanding of the microscopic world resulted in a restrictive vocabulary choice for the coverage of the biological elements: the prohibition against "bacteriological" methods of warfare could unfortunately be read as being inapplicable to later discovered (but potentially even more threatening) nonbacterial (but still biological) microorganisms such as viruses, fungi, and rickettsias.

Efforts to plug these gaps in the Geneva Protocol proved unavailing, and the buildup—both in quantity and quality—of countries' poison arsenals continued unabated. Perhaps inevitably, *use* of the despised chemicals, including use that was in blatant violation of the terms of the protocol, soon followed. Fascist Italy invaded Ethiopia in 1935, and employed CW (principally mustard gas) widely and effectively against Haile Selassie's unprotected subjects. Later, Japan applied chemicals with similar impunity against China.

But, surprisingly, the combatants for the most part avoided invoking chemical weaponry in the central battlefields of World War II, despite strong, frequent temptation to do so; despite their mutual expectation that the other side might abruptly initiate CW use at any time; despite the detailed planning and preparations for applying poisons in the battlefield; and despite the fact that all partisans were eventually massively armed with chemicals, including, in the case of Germany, with a new generation of exceptionally deadly "nerve agents" such as the notorious tabun and sarin. A combination of deterrence (the fear that the other side would retaliate in kind) and disgust (including Hitler's own distaste for using chemical weapons in formal combat—perhaps born of his own incapacitating exposure to mustard gas as a corporal during World War I) seems to have kept the European battlefields relatively "clean."

Similar patterns—albeit less pronounced—emerged with respect to biological weapons during this period, with each side relying on strategies of deterrence, preparedness, and self-restraint. Each combatant feared that its enemies might precipitously invoke biological warfare at key moments, either on the formal battlefield or in a sabotage attack behind the lines. The Allies worried especially that Nazi V-1 and V-2 rockets laden with anthrax or botulinus toxin could be targeted against England and that Japanese hot air balloons could carry anticrop or antipersonnel agents to the West Coast of the United States. Each combatant (with the curious exception of Germany) extensively researched possible offensive BW developments, as well as anti-BW defensive systems. The Americans and the British collaboratively or separately pursued a dozen potential biological agents, actively developing two that could be employed directly against humans (anthrax, which was eventually produced for the active stockpile, and botulinus toxin), as well as several others that could have been deployed against Japanese rice and other crops to hasten the country's collapse near the end of the war.

The United States's BW enterprise, personally approved (but without much enthusiasm, curiosity, or follow-up) by President Franklin Roosevelt, secretly assembled a staff of some 4,000 people and a budget of $60 million.[14] The program led to the construction of impressive facilities in Maryland, Indiana, Mississippi, and Utah, and it leveraged that investment by contracting with private academic researchers at twenty-eight universities. In 1944, the Army's Chemical Warfare Service advocated gearing up to produce as many as 275,000 botulin bombs or one million anthrax bombs per month.[15]

Although not much offensive BW material was available until late in the war, there was considerable discussion about the feasibility and strategic utility of BW use, especially against Japan, to ameliorate the costly "island hopping" process at the end of the Pacific campaign. And, in contrast to his statements pledging never to be the first to use chemical weapons, President Roosevelt never committed to eschewing the initiation of biological warfare. But the concept was always rejected, usually on the grounds that it would be more effective to devote the necessary resources (scarce air power and logistics support) to conventional bombing. While many military and civilian leaders felt they would have had to think long and hard about the moral consequences of unleashing biological warfare, President Harry Truman professed no particular ethical squeamishness about that prospect; compared to his decision to use the atomic bomb, he later implied, all other types of weapons would be morally far less problematic.

The British weaponeers went one step beyond their American counterparts, by extensively testing and stockpiling quantities of live anthrax weapons. Some five million anthrax-spiked "cattle cakes" for Nazi livestock were manufactured with the possibility of air-dropping them into Germany. Likewise, scientists at the Porton Down facility investigated the feasibility of aerial release of anthrax spores. Gruinard Island, an isolated speck off the northwest coast of Scotland, was so contaminated as a result of prolonged testing of these capabilities in 1942 to 1943, largely against tethered sheep, that it was still deemed uninhabitable and off limits some forty years later.

A handful of small-scale incidents of BW use in Europe during World War II have been claimed, but few details are available. Erhard Geissler reports that twenty-five biological sabotage operations were conducted in 1943 alone by Polish and Soviet resistance movements, but little corroborating evidence is available.[16] In one episode, the Polish underground used typhoid fever microbes to kill "a few hundred" German soldiers and Gestapo agents; the American Joint Chiefs of Staff were informed about the incident but considered that such an isolated event would not likely destroy the main taboo against BW. Likewise, the Czech resistance movement spread anthrax germs with some success on envelopes to be used by the Nazi occupying force. And it has been suggested that Soviet defenders of Stalingrad in 1942 employed a tularemia weapon against the oncoming German panzer corps, before a sudden shift in the winds, or contaminated rodents passing through the battle lines, wound up infecting far more Russians than Germans. Other similar BW-related occurrences in this era have also been described but not fully substantiated.

Japan's wartime application of biological weapons in China deserves particular mention.[17] The Japanese Army's infamous Special Unit 731, led by army surgeon Lieutenant General Shiro Ishii, not only conducted a sustained series of macabre "experiments" with BW on at least 3,000 unwilling civilian natives and prisoners of war, it also undertook full-scale local military campaigns with unconventional biological weaponry against eleven cities in the Congshan region of Manchuria—the only confirmed use of such arms in international combat in modern times. Agents included not only smallpox but also bubonic plague, anthrax, typhus, and others; incredible brutality was exhibited in the pursuit of "scientific" information and military conquest. Through it all, some temporary or tactical successes were registered, but no significant military advantage was apparently gained.

At the end of the war, American occupation forces concluded a grisly bargain: in return for relieving Ishii and some of his top associates from exposure to war crimes prosecutions, the Japanese turned over to U.S. forces the secret findings from the unspeakable procedures. Only in recent years has the full legacy of these atrocities finally begun to be revealed; moreover, some of the Japanese machinery that produced the lethal agents is still in Congshan, awaiting final cleanup and disposal.

COLD WAR ERA

After World War II, the United States, the Soviet Union, and others left no stone unturned in their reciprocal, largely offsetting, search for new military tools, and a great flowering occurred in both chemical and biological weaponry, as with many other types of armaments. The United States, for example, produced an enormous reservoir of chemical ordnance of various sorts, eventually retaining some 30,000 tons of selected CW agents for the enduring stockpile; the Soviet Union topped that figure.[18]

Regarding biological weapons, similar inventiveness and determination were demonstrated. The U.S. Army became the lead agency for the federal government's BW investigations, but the Air Force, the Navy, and the CIA participated, too, and human, animal, and plant pathogens and toxins were all explored. Testing at Dugway Proving Ground in Utah, and elsewhere throughout and even outside the continental United States, may have included thousands of open-air releases, with lethal agents such as brucellosis, tularemia, plague, and Q fever —despite a growing sense of repugnance with such ordnance.

Shockingly, some of these tests also included experiments (with supposedly benign simulants) in major American cities, exposing unsuspecting and unconsenting Americans as subjects in the explorations of BW capabilities. From 1951 through 1969 the program flourished, and various insect and rodent vectors, as well as mechanical dispersal systems, were investigated, refined, and sometimes perfected. The testing procedures, however, were often far from perfect: accidental or uncontrolled discharges sometimes unleashed lethal chemical and biological substances upon an unprepared and vulnerable public.

By 1969, the United States had stockpiled 40,000 liters of antipersonnel BW agents, 45,000 toxin-containing bullets and shrapnel bombs, and five tons of antiplant BW agents.[19] No fewer than thirty-five viable combinations of BW agents were generated, including novel and antibiotic-resistant types of pathogens.[20] Variola, in particular, was weaponized: "We made a beautiful powder for smallpox," one U.S. biological weapons officer recalled, adding "We used chemicals to protect it during dissemination and aerosolization" to spread the virus more effectively.[21]

Even after President Nixon terminated America's offensive BW program in 1969 (see below), work on the defensive side of the ledger continued apace. The United States sustained a significant biological weapons infrastructure, conducted a robust program of investigations into protective and prophylactic measures, and continued to operate capable facilities. In the 1980s, the defensive BW program intensified, with over one hundred government, university, and corporate laboratories conducting biotechnology projects for military applications. In some cases, inevitably, the ambiguous dividing line between "offensive" and "defensive" work was approached, if not crossed; critics alleged that the Department of Defense risked provoking a new BW arms race, by undertaking genetic research and development programs under the guise of inquiries into vaccines and protections.

Into the twenty-first century, similar concerns have been vetted. Secret military research, ostensibly aimed at developing countermeasures against Russian or other biological weapons, reached provocative new levels, as the Pentagon and the CIA (a) sought to develop a genetically engineered variant of anthrax (copying one purportedly developed by the USSR and now perhaps available on the international black market) in order to assess the efficacy of American vaccination efforts; (b) built and tested a model of a Soviet-era germ delivery system that might still be accessible to rogue states or terrorists; and (c) assembled a simulated BW factory, entirely from commercially available materials, to demonstrate how readily enemies could acquire the ability to mass-produce the dangerous pathogens. While the motivation behind these measures was asserted to be entirely "defensive," that is, confirming or improving the measures that would protect America from a biological attack, commentators noted that the United States would protest vociferously if any other state undertook such a substantial, ambitious, and secret BW-related program.

Moreover, just as we have now learned (as discussed below) that the Soviet/Russian chemical and biological institutions continued their offense-oriented effort long after their civilian leadership had ordered it halted, it also appears that the U.S. Central Intelligence Agency continued to maintain an inventory of lethal offensive BW agents and disseminating systems, for a period of years after the president had directly ordered their elimination.[22]

Today, the centerpiece of America's military biological weapons defense readiness program is the U.S. Army Medical Research Institute of Infectious Diseases (USAMRIID), in Fort Detrick, near Frederick, Maryland. At this site, the government sponsors a wide range of inquiries into biological pathogens, pursuing vaccines, therapies, and other measures that could aid in the fight against either biological warfare or natural disease outbreaks. The institute houses one of the few biosafety level 4 laboratories and hospitals in the world, capable of handling the most noxious substances in tight security.

The other institution critical to the U.S. side of this story is the Centers for Disease Control and Prevention (CDC) in Atlanta, Georgia, one of only two WHO "collaborating centers" authorized to house an inventory of the variola virus. The CDC undertakes basic research programs into all manner of deadly microorganisms. As is appropriate, it has instituted multiple programs to ensure protection of the variola samples and the other, even more lethal, substances it houses. But the range of natural and human threats is broad: hurricanes, earthquakes, and floods; deliberate and accidental airplane crashes; and human error on the part of even the most skilled microbiologists. Recent incidents have reestablished the U.S. government's vulnerability to high-level espionage, sabotage, incompetence, terrorism, and "brain drain."

SOVIET AND RUSSIAN PROGRAMS

The Soviet Union was regarded (at least by Western defense and intelligence authorities) as having integrated the possibility of chemical and biological warfare into its procurement, training, and combat doctrine in a much more detailed and comprehensive way than had the United States and NATO. Soviet and Warsaw Pact troops were said to be far better instructed and equipped to fight in a contaminated environment, and the impressive cadre of Chemical Troops (also responsible for biological weapons matters) was engaged in developing and testing the most sophisticated CBW agents, dispersal mechanisms, protective gear, reconnaissance capabilities, and decontamination methods.

In recent years, first glasnost, then defectors, and subsequently the emergence of democracy have allowed hordes of weapons secrets to tumble out of formerly tightly restricted Soviet archives. Western authorities have gained greater (but still incomplete) insight into two related (somewhat redundant, often feuding) Soviet cold war BW enterprises.[23] One, overtly military controlled, dates back to the 1920s and orchestrated a full panoply of Ministry of Defense activities such as BW laboratories, testing sites, and production—perhaps 30,000 people were engaged in the program, and tons of smallpox, anthrax, plague, and other deadly agents were generated annually.

The other shadow Soviet BW bureaucracy, created in 1973, proceeded in equal secrecy but under the guise of a civilian enterprise, known as Biopreparat. Using the cover of a program dedicated to medical or pharmaceutical investigations, Biopreparat developed the largest, most diverse, and most sophisticated offensive and defensive BW complex in the world—and continued operating that empire well after Moscow's adherence to the Biological Weapons Convention had rendered it illegal. The Biopreparat archipelago embraced nearly forty facilities across the country, which varied in the mixture of civilian and military work conducted. At its height in the late 1980s, the program reportedly employed approximately 30,000 scientists, engineers, and technicians on biological weapons projects, and commanded an annual budget equivalent to perhaps $1 billion.[24]

Today, the flagship of the Biopreparat cluster is the Russian State Research Center of Virology and Biotechnology, known as Vector, in Koltsovo, near Novosibirsk, in southern Siberia. Vector (along with the U.S. CDC) is one of the two WHO "collaborating centers," approved as locations for the continued storage of and experimentation on variola virus. The Soviet/Russian smallpox stocks had been initially assigned to a WHO-authorized center at the Ivanovsky Institute for Viral Preparations in Moscow. But they were abruptly and secretly transferred to Vector in 1994—allegedly because better security precautions could be undertaken to protect the virus in Koltsovo,[25] but perhaps also because the presence of a legitimate variola inventory at Vector could help provide cover for covert smallpox-related weapons research that had been under way there for years.[26] Eventually, the WHO ratified the transfer after the fact, but, of course, did not authorize or inspect any offensive BW-related work surreptitiously undertaken by Vector.

According to Ken Alibek, a defector previously engaged as deputy director at some of the most sensitive Soviet BW operations, Biopreparat and the Ministry of Defense both considered smallpox to be their "number one strategic weapon."[27] While diverse parts of the underground apparatus were experimenting with, perfecting, and mass-producing other bioweapons, including anthrax, plague, tularemia, and Ebola, the variola virus remained a focus of special interest, dating back to the WHO's global smallpox eradication campaign. Through sustained, covert research work from the 1960s through the 1980s, the Soviets not only accumulated a voluminous stockpile of ready-to-use variola virus weapons but also handcrafted an improved, genetically altered version of variola that offered greater lethality, quicker infectivity, and vaccine resistance. Facilities and inventory were updated and expanded into the 1990s.

Researchers at Vector, collaborating with three other laboratories, secretly pursued perfecting and weaponizing the variola BW. Some twenty tons of the novel liquid agent were stockpiled in the 1970s, specifically for long-range, strategic attack against the United States, Great Britain, and other European countries. (The contagiousness and high mortality rates of smallpox deterred any possible use closer to the Soviet homeland.) The USSR dedicated to this mission several of its largest intercontinental-range ballistic missiles (ICBMs): the SS-18 (previously devoted exclusively to nuclear arms) was capable of depositing 375 kilograms of viral materials, sufficient to blanket one hundred square kilometers. Since the liquid smallpox agent had a potent shelf life of a year or less, there was a requirement for continuous production at the Ministry of Defense facility at Zagorsk (now Sergiev Posad), near Moscow. Live variola agent could be transferred from storage tanks into cluster bomblets, cruise missiles, or other ordnance in only two or three days.

The Soviet operation conducted open-air testing of live BW agents and weapons on Vozrozhdeniye ("Rebirth") Island in the Aral Sea (in what is now Kazakhstan and Uzbekistan). The field tests began there as early as 1936 and continued unabated until the site was closed in 1992—all with disastrous consequences for the local and regional environment. Smallpox, anthrax, and all manner of other noxious BW arms, developed by the Ministry of Defense or by Biopreparat, were tested by a staff of 150 scientists, technicians, and soldiers, on laboratory animals, livestock, and plants, in order to design agents less susceptible to the deleterious effects of heat, light, radiation, and antibiotics. Now, as the water level of the Aral Sea continues to drop precipitously (a consequence of misbegotten irrigation engineering), the island expands and thus grows closer to the mainland, bringing its buried cache of weapons, spores, and other BW detritus ever closer to civilian populations and uncontrollable animal vectors on the mainland.

Other countries, too, pursued covert BW and CW capabilities throughout the cold war era, as detailed further below. There were occasional credible allegations about the exercise of these arsenals, such as Egypt's use of CW during its intervention in the Yemeni Civil War of 1963 to 1967 and Libya's CW applications against Chad in 1986 to 1987. There were even allegations, readily dismissed as frivolous, that the United States used biological weaponry against North Korea in 1952, and there have been repeated claims by Cuba, again without the benefit of much proof, of American BW efforts against the Castro regime.

BIOLOGICAL WEAPONS AGENTS TODAY

The bounty of nature and the inventiveness of humankind have combined to offer the world a tragically wide array of potential biological weapons. Any complete survey is beyond the scope of this book: one international group of experts identified sixty-seven pathogens and forty-eight toxins of concern for biological warfare purposes, and that list specified only the antihuman agents, not those targeting plants or animals.[28] Ninety-seven substances of widespread concern are listed by the Australia Group, economically developed countries who meet to coordinate their export control regimes related to BW and CW proliferation. [29] Still, brief note of some of the highlights can provide a glimpse into the multiple threats that security, arms control, and public health experts must confront.

The military list of the world's potential viral killers would surely feature, in addition to variola, the viruses that cause varieties of encephalitis, psittacosis, yellow fever, and strains of influenza, as well as the newly emerging hemorrhagic fever viruses such as Ebola, hantavirus, and Marburg. Bacterial agents include the microbes responsible for anthrax, plague, tularemia (rabbit fever), glanders, cholera, typhoid fever, and meningitis. The leading rickettsia would be Rocky Mountain spotted fever. Toxin weapons could consist of botulinum, saxitoxin (a strong neurotoxin), and those drawn from castor beans (ricin), cobra or rattlesnake venom, scorpions, and shellfish. Adding to the noxious roster those agents usually intended to incapacitate, rather than to kill, would contribute Q fever, brucellosis, salmonella, and dengue virus. Expanding the inventory to incorporate antiplant and antianimal pathogens, we would list rice blast, stem rust, tobacco mosaic virus, foot-and-mouth disease, and rinderpest, among others.

More telling than the diversity of these microbes is their power. Botulinum toxin, for example, has been described as "the most lethal substance known"— only tenths of a microgram would be deadly, and it is said to be thousands or hundreds of thousands of times more lethal than the best CW nerve agents.[30] Although careful, thorough studies have never been conducted of the effects of many of these agents, the spare record (coupled with anecdotal evidence and scale modeling) suggests that pound-for-pound (or dollar-for-dollar), biological weapons are much more dangerous than the other "weapons of mass destruction," nuclear arms, or chemical agents.

That potential lethality has not been lost on defense experts. Colin Powell, U.S. Secretary of State and former Chair of the Joint Chiefs of Staff, remarked after the Persian Gulf War that "of all the various weapons of mass destruction, biological weapons are of the greatest concern to me."[31] These weapons, usually arriving in colorless, odorless vapors, may initiate an infection in a person that might not be revealed for days and may never be recognized as the action of a hostile force.

Of course, a variety of other characteristics, beyond lethality rates, would combine to define an optimal biological weapon. Planners would look to the hardiness of each candidate agent, to assess its survivability in sunlight, rain, or heat; the speed of transmission (both the time lag between exposure and illness for a particular individual and the rate of passage through a targeted community); the existence of adequate diagnostic techniques, treatment regimens, and vaccines for the defense; the ease of mass production, storage, and weaponization; and other factors. But the potential power of this dysfunctional family of hostile biological agents is large, impressive, and quite depressing.

DIFFERENTIATING CHEMICAL
AND BIOLOGICAL WEAPONS

Gradually through the post–World War II era, the story of chemical weapons and the story of biological weapons began to diverge. Militarily, chemical weapons were seen (at least by some) as retaining potential utility: there were arguments (largely rejected in the West, but even so, one could see their plausibility) about scenarios in which chemical rounds might carry some local tactical advantage. Even if not fully decisive, deft application of chemicals, it was thought, would make everything tougher for the enemy, confounding ordinary communications, movement, and logistics. Moreover, the imperative of deterring the other side's invocation of its massive CW seemed to rest upon the threat of retaliation "in kind": we had to match them, if not shell for shell, at least in some rough aggregate of chemical capability. Finally, verification of compliance with any CW control regime appeared to pose insurmountable difficulties, given the "dual-use" phenomenon (the inescapable fact that many of the same substances, facilities, and equipment used to produce chemical arms were simultaneously useful in producing important civilian products) and the ubiquitous employment throughout the national civilian economy of chemical compounds that could inherently carry profound weapons applications.

Biological weaponry, in contrast, was increasingly deemed unusable; it was too uncontrollable, too unpredictable. Its dispersion patterns, its concentrations, and its effectiveness could vary radically with local weather conditions; it might waft into unprotected civilian areas or boomerang back onto the user's own troops and territory. And uncontrolled infectivity threatened everyone, at a time when no country could be confident of its ability to withstand various sorts of human, plant, or animal epidemics. Moreover, most known BW agents acted slowly on an individual and spread slowly to others, making it difficult to deliver a timely military blow. Also, defenses against BW attack seemed feasible: if the enemy troops were forewarned, they could be vaccinated, shielded, and otherwise prepared. Thus, despite extensive experimentation and testing, there was no known "perfect" biological weapon agent, and there did not seem to be a suitable military niche for BW in the modern defense arsenal.

It was, instead, increasingly feared that continued biological weapons inventiveness by the United States, the Soviet Union, and a few others was threatening to lead the world toward the production of new generations of germ armaments whose principal application would eventually be by "nonstate actors." Those terrorists might adapt the military understandings into inexpensive, crude—but still effective—BW devices with which they could harm, threaten, or hold hostage unprotected civilian populations.

The international diplomatic proceedings largely took their cue from this refined military and political attitude, and the question of global control over BW was increasingly (although not without controversy) split off from the issue of CW. While earnest efforts still continued to extend the reach of the 1925 Geneva Protocol to deal more effectively with both categories of ordnance together, a companion enterprise was also launched to negotiate a separate instrument, to be focused exclusively on the seemingly more tractable problem of BW. Although France, the Soviet Union, and others resisted—arguing that any effort to carve out biological weapons for special treatment might have the perverse effect of licensing and thereby stimulating an even greater race to pursue chemical weapons—many pragmatists were eventually attracted to dealing with whatever portions of the overall disarmament problem seemed amenable to prompt resolution.

A major impetus came from the United States, where President Richard Nixon declared on November 25, 1969, that America was renouncing bacteriological and biological methods of warfare, unilaterally destroying its existing stockpile of offensive biological weapons and agents, and closing all its facilities engaged in the production of offensive BW materials. On February 14, 1970, the White House announced that the ban would be extended to cover toxins as well.

With that unexpected leadership, the pace of the international negotiations quickened. By March 1971, the Soviet Union had reversed its diplomatic position, agreeing to the concept of promptly articulating a separate BW convention; by August of that year, there was a jointly agreed treaty text tabled by the two superpowers; by December, the United Nations General Assembly had approved the draft by a vote of 110 to 0. The Convention on the Prohibition of the Development, Production, and Stockpiling of Bacteriological (Biological) and Toxin Weapons and on Their Destruction (commonly referred to as the Biological Weapons Convention or BWC) was opened for signature on April 10, 1972, and it entered into force on March 26, 1975. Today, it has attracted some 144 parties, including all five permanent members of the United Nations Security Council, as well as most of the countries of major proliferation concern, such as Iran, Iraq, Libya, and North Korea. Notable "holdout" countries still include Israel, Egypt, Syria, Sudan, and Algeria.

In many respects, the BWC is a significant improvement over its predecessor, the Geneva Protocol. For example, the BWC is much more aggressive in its choice of verbs, enjoining its countries "never in any circumstances to develop, produce, stockpile, or otherwise acquire or retain" biological weapons agents or toxins, or the means for hostile delivery of them.[32] (The BWC does not explicitly bar the *use* of such weapons, on the diplomatic principle that the Geneva Protocol had already accomplished at least that much, as well as on the logical principle that no country could use BW agents unless it had already violated the proscriptions against *possessing* them in the first place.) The BWC also deserves credit for including the full range of biological threats, both known and unknown: it proscribes "microbial or other biological agents, or toxins whatever their origin or method of production,"[33] and its title uses the terms *biological* and *bacteriological* interchangeably, to demonstrate that all varieties of microorganisms are embraced.

Nonetheless, the BWC also suffers shortcomings all too familiar to its predecessor. The treaty's spare five pages contain essentially no verification provisions to ensure compliance: it incorporates no inspection or even data-reporting procedures. Likewise, the accord lacks modern enforcement or sanctions mechanisms; it specifies only a rudimentary process for resolving ambiguities and adjudicating compliance controversies. Largely because of the negotiation context—the United States was proceeding with unilateral BW disarmament anyway, independent of anything that other states might do in the area—the diplomats thought they could afford to be relatively relaxed about those niceties. They concentrated instead on the basic "ban" provisions of the treaty, failing to demonstrate what subsequently became a necessary and now reflexive fastidiousness about verification procedures.

Just as important, the BWC negotiators were satisfied with a set of treaty commitments that allowed biological agent development, production, and permanent possession as long as those activities were confined to types and quantities justified for "prophylactic, protective, or other peaceful purposes."[34] This loophole means that inquiries into BW defenses (e.g., "gas masks" and other protective clothing, sensors that could detect and identify airborne pathogens) are permitted, to allow a country to gird itself against the threat of another state's offensive BW attack. But the distinction between "offensive" and "defensive" work can be elusive: a country might need to retain a certain quantity of diverse active lethal agents and BW delivery vehicles, in order to test the efficacy of its prophylaxis routines. Unfortunately, such a practice carries an inherent offensive capability, because even a modest experimental offensive arsenal might be quickly multiplied to become a significant offensive force. By that same token, one could justify research on *new* types of potential BW agents, on the grounds that only by keeping fully current with possible breakthroughs in BW offenses could one be certain about the ongoing adequacy of one's own defenses.

In a similar vein, the BWC authorizes and encourages its parties to proceed with research into "peaceful uses" of biological agents, such as the pursuit of improved pharmaceuticals and hybrid crops. The negotiators recognized the potential for scientific advancement in such areas, and they were at pains not to inhibit that inventiveness and even to promote international cooperation in pursuit of it. But the dual capability of so many biological substances, processes, and types of equipment and facilities generates unavoidable complications for a weapons control regime. Some biological agents can be adapted for both peaceful and military applications; some techniques developed for civilian purposes can cross over into weapons work (and vice versa). Some buildings and equipment can have multiple functions and may be cleaned up and converted from weapons to nonweapons applications (and perhaps back again) relatively quickly. There is usually no way to confine the information obtained through basic research or to guard against its conversion to hostile purposes—at least not without intrusive inspection and other verification arrangements that the BWC parties were unwilling to countenance in 1972.

BWC COMPLIANCE CONTROVERSIES

Despite those apprehensions, the Biological Weapons Convention attracted global support and widespread adherence. The entire issue of BW largely (if only momentarily) slipped off the world's "radar screen," as most people considered the treaty to be an adequate solution to a potential weapons problem that—due to its own military shortcomings—never attained the virulence people had long feared.

Any complacency on that score, however, was short-lived. Doubts or ambiguities about treaty compliance quickly arose, as the United States challenged the Soviet Union's conformity to the most fundamental BWC obligations, and two sustained controversies—both pitting Washington, D.C., against Moscow in some of the most harsh, direct, and protracted cold war confrontations—soon embroiled the treaty.

The first dispute resulted from an outbreak in April 1979 of anthrax illnesses near the large Siberian city of Sverdlovsk (now known by its pre-Communist name, Yekaterinburg). American authorities feared that the eruption—with illnesses and fatalities reportedly numbering in the thousands—may have been triggered by an accident at a secret military installation in the city, a facility long suspected of engaging in covert offensive biological weapons production in violation of the BWC.[35] When pressed on the issue, Soviet authorities stonewalled, asserting simply that anthrax was endemic to the region—there had periodically been notorious natural outbreaks—and that this particular round of the disease had been caused by the sale and consumption of contaminated black market beef. The controversy was joined, however, when American experts concluded by indirect observation that the type of anthrax encountered in the incident was more likely the variety spread by inhalation (e.g., exposure to a toxic cloud suddenly released from an industrial accident), rather than by ingestion. Furthermore, evidence began to mount that the scale of the outbreak, the responsive measures adopted by local officials to combat it, and the geographic dispersion pattern of the victims (principally fanning downwind from the suspect facility) were all inconsistent with the official Soviet explanation.

The controversy raged for years, with the United States charging that the Soviet Union had engaged in a direct, sustained violation of the BWC, and with Moscow just as insistently denying it. As the issue festered through the 1980s, the BWC itself fell into some disrepute, as the inadequacy of its verification and dispute-resolution procedures became more pronounced. Only in the 1990s was the veil partially lifted, when newly elected President Boris Yeltsin (who had been the Communist Party chairman for Sverdlovsk at the time of the accident) publicly admitted that the Soviet Union had retained an illegal offensive biological weapons program and that the Sverdlovsk outbreak in 1979 had been the result of a tragic mishap at the BW facility there. Even so, some important questions about the issue have still not been entirely answered, and the implications for the BWC and for biological weapons activities more generally have not been fully sorted out.

The other BWC-related compliance incident, or set of related incidents, arising at about the same time, also remains somewhat murky. Beginning in the late 1970s, reports began filtering out of Laos about targeting of the rebellious H'Mong mountain tribes by air-dropped toxins that (at least sometimes) appeared as a "yellow rain" emitted by government aircraft. People splattered by the substance reported a variety of illnesses, from nausea to dizziness to internal bleeding; some were said to have died from it. In 1978, comparable allegations emerged from Kampuchea (Cambodia), following the invasion by Vietnam. And in 1980, there were strikingly similar assertions about Soviet use of air-dropped poisons against the mujahideen rebels in Afghanistan.[36]

In each case, the initial suspicions gave rise to persistent refugee reports, then to sporadic international inquiries and abrupt responses, then to largely abortive attempts at authoritative on-site inspections, then to widely circulated public allegations, and eventually to vigorous international recriminations. The United States at length obtained a leaf sample from Laos, spotted with a yellow goo; some laboratory analysts identified it as being laced with tricothecene, a strongly hazardous mycotoxin (a fungus- or mold-based poison), whose use as a weapon would be inconsistent with both the Geneva Protocol and the Biological Weapons Convention. The American government formally alleged that the Soviet Union, directly or via Vietnamese proxies, had engaged in illegal poison war-making.

Critics argued, however, that the U.S. government's case was flawed from the beginning. Even the single "smoking gun" leaf sample was capable of alternative explanations—in particular, the "yellow rain" could have been entirely natural in origin, resulting from local honeybees engaging in massive cleansing defecation flights. The other evidence was similarly equivocal, and neither side was able to assemble a fully persuasive case in the "court of world public opinion." The Soviets and their allies, for their part, consistently denied all the allegations, but only in the most conclusory fashion, and they declined to offer probative exculpatory evidence.

The behavior—or at least the reports about toxic chemicals—largely terminated after 1984, and competing explanations (possible Soviet use of nonlethal smoke to disguise aerial operations, or hypothetical Vietnamese application of some of the herbicides and nonlethal riot control agents they had earlier captured from the Americans) still abound. The impact of the event on the fighting in Southeast and Southwest Asia was surely minor, within the context of those wars, but the political impact on controlling chemical and biological weaponry, and on the viability of the BWC, was profound.

Deep skepticism about Soviet, and now Russian, compliance with the obligations of the Biological Weapons Convention has persisted beyond those two particular flash points. Some of the debate now focuses on the possible role of the national leadership: "What did they know and when did they know it?" That is, were Presidents Gorbachev and Yeltsin witting accomplices to what are now widely acknowledged as continuing violations of the BWC, were they kept ignorant of the violations by rogue subordinates, or did they connive to maintain "plausible deniability" while allowing the underground activity to persist?

The behind-the-scenes dealings inside the Kremlin over the years have remained shrouded in mystery. Dissidents claim that Gorbachev had explicitly approved at least the broad parameters of a $1 billion illicit BW program—with an ever-widening roster of agents being developed as part of an expanding bioinfrastructure—beginning in 1985, at the same time that he was assuring his Western interlocutors that the violations had been cleaned up. Smallpox was allegedly highlighted as a "special item" on the general secretary's list of diseases to pursue, and a huge new viral reactor was approved for the Vector facility to speed the processing of variola for patently offensive purposes.

In 1992, Yeltsin issued a decree reaffirming Russia's commitment to the BWC and reasserting central control over all federal biological weapons-related activities. He undertook to slash the number of personnel involved in the program by 50 percent and the research funding by 30 percent, to terminate all offensive BW research, to dissolve the Ministry of Defense office responsible for the offensive BW program, and to investigate activities at other suspect sites. Still, outsiders worried that even if Yeltsin were fully sincere in his effort to oust the entrenched BW enterprise, he might have lacked the political clout to tear down the established interests or the detailed knowledge about the interstices of the BW nodes to root out all aspects of the program. Even today, suspicions linger about what well-cloaked weapons-related activity might still be occurring in concealed corners of the Vector installation.[37]

It does appear that many previously hostile BW facilities have been closed in recent years, and a substantial "conversion" operation has been undertaken, with Biopreparat facilities—led by the Vector lab in Koltsovo—lurching toward sustainable civilian employment. A modicum of financial assistance from the United States, via the Nunn-Lugar Cooperative Threat Reduction program and other vehicles, has facilitated this transformation, although critics complain about the paltry size and restrictive conditions of the U.S. efforts to assist the remnants of the former Soviet Union in transforming themselves into modern, civilian-controlled states. While most of this American seed money has concentrated on nuclear weapons, with the highest priority tasks being to facilitate improvements in the management, accounting, control, safety, and reduction of the former Soviet Union's nuclear arsenal, substantial attention has been paid to chemical and biological weapons matters, too.

Smallpox has been a focus of the U.S. contribution, as the Departments of Defense and Health and Human Services have reviewed $5 million worth of proposed counterterrorism projects from Vector concerning (1) recognition and diagnosis of the disease, (2) pathogenesis, and (3) development of a new antiviral drug for smallpox victims.[38] Upgrading physical security and converting former CW/BW personnel and institutions to civilian employment have been stressed. Vector's director, Lev S. Sandakhchiev, has welcomed a steady stream of foreign visitors and inspectors and has undertaken a growing, remunerative agenda of joint research and development enterprises with Western firms in commercial areas involving medicines, cosmetics, and other ventures.

Reduced to a staff of 2,200 scientists and technicians (less than half its previous complement), Vector has abandoned or converted many of its weapons-related facilities. "Dozens" of installations approved as recently as the Gorbachev era for conducting further work on an offensive smallpox weapon capability now stand empty, unfinished, and deteriorating.[39] Variola work continues, but, it is said, only in the effort to develop improved vaccines and to glean greater understanding of the fundamentals of virulence and immunology.[40] Still, much of the human capital remains intact: the knowledge extracted from years of aggressive variola BW-related research lingers, potentially available for either weapons purposes or more benign applications. And some doubters remain concerned that retrograde elements in the Russian bureaucracy may not have totally abandoned their Soviet-era offensive BW conceits.

ROGUE STATE THREATS

Throughout the cold war years, the world also had to deal with the notion that biological and chemical weaponry might also hold an irresistible appeal for a range of unstable, provocative "rogue" countries. Today, even as the superpowers have ostentatiously renounced any need to sustain their own massive inventories of BW and CW, the dangers posed by further proliferation have, if anything, accelerated. In 1992, the president of the United Nations Security Council declared on behalf of the members that the proliferation of weapons of mass destruction constituted a "threat to the peace" sufficient to invoke the Security Council's extraordinary powers under chapter VII of the UN Charter. In the same vein, President Clinton in 1994 declared a state of national emergency relating to the spread of weapons of mass destruction, asserting that the potential use of biological, chemical, or nuclear weapons by a terrorist group or a rogue state constitutes "an unusual and extraordinary threat to the national security, foreign policy, and economy of the United States."[41]

The historical record validates these concerns, demonstrating that the proscriptions against acquisition and use of unconventional weapons are no more airtight today than previously. Iraq certainly applied chemical ordnance, with virtual impunity, against its Kurdish minority population in 1987 to 1988, and on a larger scale and for a longer duration, in its war against Iran. On a smaller magnitude, Iran retaliated with CW of its own, and both sides escaped any effective international condemnation for their actions. There have also been allegations, far from established, that Iraq used smallpox or other biological weapons against Iran in that conflict and inoculated its own soldiers against variola as a precaution.[42]

Also noteworthy is the experience of the Gulf War, in which Iraq prepared but did not employ its estimable chemical capabilities. In the aftermath of that conflict, we have realized that Baghdad also had a significant biological weapons program—perhaps as much as one ton of active agents. After years of "cat and mouse" games with United Nations inspectors, Iraq finally admitted to producing 500,000 liters of BW materials, including significant quantities of anthrax, botulinum toxin, ricin, camel pox virus, and aflatoxin (a type of carcinogenic mycotoxin). It deployed twenty-five Al Hussein SCUD missiles and 160 aircraft bombs loaded with the deadly substances in four locations. Dozens of truck-mounted BW-capable aerosol launchers may also have been deployed to the front lines. The plan (at least until allied coalition forces secured full air superiority in the early days of the conflict) had been to spray the lethal mixture on liberating forces moving up from Saudi Arabia in the south. According to some calculations, Iraq's accumulation of botulinum toxin alone would have been sufficient, if perfectly disseminated, to kill fifteen billion people.[43]

American leaders were apprehensive about what Iraq's invocation of BW could have meant on the battlefield and in cities within striking distance; it was often cited as the most dangerous and provocative scenario Baghdad could pursue. In the end, Saddam Hussein seems to have been deterred from selecting a BW or CW option by a combination of coalition preparedness (including vaccinating 100,000 U.S. troops against anthrax and another 8,000 against botulism toxin—the two main suspected Iraqi BW agents) and implicit, but unmistakable, threats of overwhelming retaliatory force.

Despite the fact that Iraq was a long-standing member of the Biological Weapons Convention, the international community was largely ignorant of the illegal offensive BW program there until UN Special Commission inspectors started poking around Saddam Hussein's facilities after the war, and especially until a prominent defector, Hussein Kamel (Saddam's son-in-law), briefly fled Iraq in 1995 and offered to spill previously unrevealed data about the massive size, location, and diversity of the country's covert BW apparatus. Even so, UN officials contend that only the tip of this particularly offensive BW iceberg has yet been revealed and that Iraq could quickly reconstitute its deadly arsenal whenever international scrutiny is relaxed. United Nations leaders note that Baghdad has been noticeably more opaque regarding its BW programs than it had been regarding chemical weapons, nuclear arms, or long-range missiles— even after many of the nonbiological weapons' hitherto secret facilities, stockpiles, and detritus had been uncovered, cataloged, and destroyed, the Iraqi biological weapons program remained shrouded in ominous mystery.

Among other "rogue" states, Libya emerged as a prominent chemical and biological weapons concern in the 1980s. After experimenting with the possibilities of CW in a border skirmish with Chad, Libya constructed a modern CBW manufacturing capability, with enormous facilities at Rabta and Tarhunah, under the guise of a purported pharmaceutical infrastructure. In 1995, reports suggested that Libya may have attempted to lure into its service some of the disaffected biological weapons experts from South Africa who had developed at least a modest lethal BW program for the apartheid regime.

If published or leaked Central Intelligence Agency reports are credited, the multilateral allure of biological armaments has never been greater. At least ten countries are deemed to possess their own secret, illegal caches of BW, to be actively pursuing forbidden offensive biological military investigations, or to be progressing rapidly in those directions.[44] In 2001, the United States publicly accused five countries—North Korea, Iraq, Iran, Libya, and Syria—of violating the Biological Weapons Convention and noted (at a conference of BWC parties) that other nations could readily be added to the illicit germ-warfare roster.[45]

Smallpox virus, in particular, may be sought—and, some fear, already obtained—by evil-minded or irresponsible rogues. North Korea, Iran, and Iraq top the list of suspects, with Libya and Syria perhaps somewhat behind in the "variola race." Other sources would add China, India, Israel, and perhaps Pakistan, Cuba, South Africa, and the Czech Republic to the roster of countries that may already have poached a variola weapon from Soviet biologists, covertly acquired and retained it through other means, or attempted to do so. While the evidence on the public record is far from conclusive, there have been such hints as blood samples from North Korean soldiers showing evidence of recent smallpox vaccination; Iraq may have vaccinated its troops, too, and manufactured additional vaccinia doses as late as 1989.

Many have concluded, therefore, that it is a mischaracterization to describe the WHO effort as a program dedicated to eradicating the "last remaining smallpox virus samples." Instead, they conclude, the most that we can undertake would be to destroy the "last *known* remaining smallpox virus samples." To pretend that we were truly accomplishing more than that, that we were in fact ridding the planet of *all* vestiges of this deadly virus would be cruelly misleading. In the words of one observer, to overadvertise what is at stake would be "to perpetrate a fraud," since the WHO lacks any real prospect of cracking open whatever secret variola caches exist in North Korea or elsewhere.[46]

In this vein, there have been proposals to label the use of biological weapons in general, or smallpox in particular, as a war crime or crime against humanity, exposing any civilian or soldier who orders or applies the germs to individual criminal prosecution, at home or in a foreign or international tribunal. Certainly, some possible applications of variola or other lethal agents would readily fit into those categories, if they were dispensed in an indiscriminate or disproportionate fashion. But some would argue that total, global eradication of variola would make a much stronger statement: any possession of the virus for any purpose would then be per se illegal, and the international norm against BW of any ilk would be strengthened.

Finally, one more modern phenomenon must be added to the roster of international BW concerns: the danger of uncontrollable Russian military/scientific "brain drain." As Russia's economy continues to falter, and as the former weapons elites are deprived of remunerative, high-status, professionally rewarding outlets for their talents, these individuals will be tempted to sell their expertise on the open (or the covert) market. A well-financed "rogue" state or terrorist cell might entice cooperation—long-term or short-term—from any of the 60,000 or so people who acquired BW competence under the regime of Biopreparat or the Soviet Ministry of Defense. Iran and other "states of concern" have invested heavily in recruiting inside the former Soviet Union; there have long been rumors that emigrants or temporary "consultants" from Russia have found their way to numerous such locales.[47]

GENETIC ENGINEERING

In any event, biological weaponry is once again a growth area for the world's competitive instincts. The nightmare scenario, no longer capable of being consigned simply to the realm of fantasy, raises fears that newly emerging viruses and some of the modern techniques of genetic engineering surveyed in chapter 2 could soon be (if they haven't already been) mated and turned to hostile purposes. The culmination of that line of inquiry would be the emergence of a new line of "designer" biological and toxin agents, surmounting many of the weaknesses that military leaders have found in "ordinary" germ weapons. Such a genetic revolution could drive, once again, the conclusion that in the long term, military competition systematically favors offenses over defenses. That is, it now seems to be a feature of nature that in biological warfare, the innovations of the aggressor (spawning new iterations of killer bugs) can routinely stay ahead of the responses of the defenders (with invention of a suitable antidote or vaccine consuming disproportionately more time and resources).

Prominent among fears would be the invocation of a chimera weapon, the name given to an artificially manufactured biological agent that would combine the worst genetic features of two (or more) diverse existing BW organisms. According to the Soviet defector Ken Alibek, Biopreparat had already succeeded in generating such chimeras, by deftly combining lethal genes from the Ebola virus, or those from another pernicious biological pest (and possible weapon), Venezuelan equine encephalitis, with those of variola or of the vaccinia virus (the close relative of variola that had been used for vaccinations and that has proven to be unusually manipulable as a vector for other genetic-engineering techniques). Critics dispute the notion that such biological cocktails were created or that they would be especially significant compared to simply inserting both types of virus into a single biological weapon. Nevertheless, tinkering with genomes supplied by nature could herald a precipitously more dangerous form of biological weapons agent.

These futuristic BW tools could, at least hypothetically, be more lethal in smaller quantities, quicker-acting, and more rapidly transmitted than existing devices. They could have a staying power (remaining viable in the soil, water, or air) greater than that of existing agents—or, if the offense's strategy so demanded, they could perhaps be crafted to have only a short "half-life" in selected climatic conditions. They could be quicker and easier to reproduce and purify. They could target humans, animals, plants, or even machines in unanticipated ways, escaping existing systems of detection, protection, and treatment. They might be so esoteric or stealthy that the target country would not recognize that it had been deliberately exposed to an imported disease or from where the vector had been launched. Some such weapons might be designed to be employed selectively, only against an enemy's top leadership, for example, rather than against the entire military or civilian population, and might have the effect of undercutting the leader's stamina, judgment, stability, or decisiveness—which might be more devastating to a war effort than would be an immediate death followed by an orderly succession. Perhaps rapacious biologists could craft an "ethnically selective" BW agent, targeting a defined population group because of some minute, unique genetic characteristic, while leaving all other races (including, presumably, the attacker's) unafflicted.

Weapons of that ilk would make "old style" biological agents obsolete, and they may not be so very far away. Research in government and private laboratories, in the United States and elsewhere, has already created new recombinant organisms, at a much greater pace than anyone had predicted. Surely the rate of human inventiveness—and the facility with which such civilian designs are adapted to military purposes—threatens to outstrip our ability to deal with the new germ weapons in a judicious manner.

TERRORIST THREATS

Subnational actors, more than regular armies, may be the immediate beneficiaries of these BW materials and emerging technologies. For terrorists, BW may be the ultimate weapon, for several reasons. First, at least some of the time, biological weapons can be cheap. The initial investment for a significant BW inventory might be as low as $10 million—some say one could set up production for as little as $10,000—and experts calculate that the "cost per fatality" of biological warfare can be much less than the comparable figures for nuclear, chemical, or conventional combat. It's not for nothing that BW frequently earns the sobriquet "the poor man's atomic bomb."[48] Second, biological agents are accessible. Some exist naturally in the wild; some may be available commercially, by theft, or on the international black market. Although variola and the most esoteric "designer" biological agents are likely to be closely guarded and hard to construct from scratch, terrorists might be satisfied with a relatively "crude" version of BW, and the raw ingredients are more plentiful than are the fissile materials necessary for nuclear devices.

Third, the facilities necessary for planning, preparing, and conducting a BW operation are relatively undemanding. The manufacturing buildings need not be large, uniquely designed, or conspicuous. The equipment need not be particularly specialized or expensive. It may not be an exaggeration to suggest that any two-car garage could be adapted for BW laboratory and production purposes without unduly raising the suspicion of the neighbors. Certainly a conventional light-industrial facility—a microbrewery or a small pharmaceutical manufacturer, for example—could be converted by a BW entrepreneur without too much expense or notice. Fourth, the job would not require an undue amount of technical expertise. While the obvious dangers of the task would require at least some experience with biohazards, a BW project may be less demanding of sustained, dedicated organizational and technical talent than some other enterprises terrorists have already undertaken.

Moreover, the "delivery system" for biological warfare imposes few rigors. A rudimentary aerial dispersal mechanism could churn out a deadly dose of pathogen for unsuspecting millions simply by flying over Washington, D.C., in a small airplane, steering a boat around Manhattan Island, or driving an open truck through the freeways of Los Angeles. Experts and journalists have already done some of the terrorists' conceptual work in this area, publishing vivid, detailed descriptions of how a secret BW incursion might be effectuated anonymously yet with devastating impact. More recently, revelations that some of the terrorists responsible for the September 11, 2001, attacks may have earlier been investigating the suitability of agricultural crop dusters as a bioterrorism device have prompted reappraisal of the technical feasibility of such a scenario, as well as augmentation of security procedures to guard against it.

Finally, the defensive systems for terrorists' targets are still underdeveloped and inadequate. America's public health infrastructure and its national security apparatus—including systems to detect bioterrorism, to recognize an anomalous disease outbreak as an attack, and to provide prompt and effective treatment and amelioration—are undergoing substantial upgrading. Still, the task of training and equipping even the local "first responders" for a potential future BW terrorist incident has not yet been adequately achieved. Particularly with a long-dormant disease such as smallpox, doctors and other community health workers are no longer accustomed to recognize the illness and—unless tipped off by exogenous sources—would have little reason to focus on that obscure possibility in making an initial diagnosis. Experts have concluded, therefore, that the scenario of a successful terrorist use of a variola weapon against the United States civilian population is all too real and immediate.

The staggering September 11, 2001, terrorist attacks—using civilian airliners as devastating flying bombs against the Pentagon and the World Trade Center towers—and their still-unraveling aftermath have provided something of a proof test of the antiterrorism system, as well as a "wake-up call from Hell" in measuring the community's strengths and weaknesses. In some respects, the report card looks pretty good: the National Guard was mobilized within minutes of the World Trade Center towers crash; the affiliations between the Centers for Disease Control and Prevention and the state and local health institutions became operational about as quickly as they could; heroism and quick action by many police and firefighters saved countless lives; and a cadre of doctors was quickly assembled, standing by to receive waves of injured victims who, tragically, never appeared.

On the other hand, the nation's response to the October 2001 wave of anthrax deliveries, threats, and hoaxes proves nothing so much as how pernicious the bioterrorism challenge really is. Still far from resolved at the time of this writing, this blast of germ attacks suddenly inflicted additional crippling shocks upon the U.S. leadership, economy, and psyche. The House and Senate office buildings in Washington, D.C., were abruptly closed down, multiple executive branch agency mailrooms were temporarily abandoned, the major media headquarters in New York were victimized, and everyone across the country began to look askance at the slightest irregularity in postal communications. President Bush had to reassure a nervous public that he did not have anthrax— and even then, he continued to obscure whether he had received prophylactic treatment against the disease. There was a spasmodic run on ciprofloxacin, the leading antianthrax medication, accompanied by worries about the adequacy of supplies. The number of false alarms and hoaxes, of course, greatly outnumbered real threats, but each incident evoked a full-fledged response, until the rather inadequate and slow testing mechanisms could verify or disprove a danger.

Confusion, delays, and distress multiplied, as the federal and local health and law enforcement institutions seemed incapable of responding with decisiveness and vigor to the growing turmoil and of communicating effectively and authoritatively about it with a profoundly spooked populace.[49] Apparently not recalling the auguries of multiple experts over the years, many are only now raising the alarm, asking "Why weren't we warned about this?" when, in fact, the literature abounds with prescient, but unheeded, forecasts. The simple, ugly fact is that there is no easy answer, no obvious response to the specter of mailed anthrax spores that are credible enough to demand a vigorous reaction and deadly enough to panic the population.

The nation's political and legal structures may also be inadequate to cope with modern international and domestic bioterrorism. The national security community is not yet organized, staffed, and trained to respond in a coherent, comprehensive manner to the alarm bells of emerging international or domestic terrorist threats. Better intelligence and threat assessment capabilities, along with improved military tools to deal effectively with nonstate actors, will be essential. The 2001 creation of a new Office of Homeland Security—while symbolizing the need to pull together diverse agency responsibilities—is no magic bullet. Bureaucratic battles over the office's statutory authority, resources, and turf must be resolved in order to effectively unite the alphabet soup of federal agencies (FBI, CIA, Federal Emergency Management Agency, CDC, Department of Defense, etc.) that must collaborate in the counterterrorism mission. The Bush administration therefore rightly warns that the multifront war against emergent terrorism will be an ongoing struggle for years to come.

Bioterrorism challenges also stress the traditional public health law standards and the framework of emergency management law and procedures. Customary state and local "police power" provisions governing quarantines, mandatory examinations and vaccinations, and other more extreme safety and sanitary conditions—crafted to deal with earlier, simpler types of outbreaks— may be insufficient to confront today's more incendiary problems. Seemingly simple questions of overlapping local, state, and federal jurisdiction and funding may confound effective collaboration on these vital efforts. A series of recent antiterrorism statutes has toughened the criminal sanctions against biological and other wanton destruction and has increased the rigor with which shipments of potentially harmful materials are scrutinized, but no one would contend that airtight restrictions are yet in place.

While there is now greater recognition of the problem, and an increased willingness to confront the novel threats, much more work (and money) will be required to put into place adequate protective measures. Although it is difficult to discern a true national antiterrorism budget because so many federal expenditures in this area are relevant for multiple purposes, generous infusions in the late 1990s probably brought this account to over $10 billion annually, and in late 2001 the Bush administration proposed an emergency supplement to bolster spending by an additional $1.5 billion. By early 2002, the ante for bioterrorism prevention alone had risen to $6 billion.[50]

Recent simulation exercises—a civilian equivalent of antiterrorism "war games"—have revealed the national bioterrorism defense inadequacies in sharp relief. A "Dark Winter" exercise, conducted in June 2001 at Andrews Air Force Base by the Center for Strategic and International Studies, the Johns Hopkins University Center for Civilian Biodefense Studies, and other nongovernmental organizations, featured a hypothetical smallpox attack against the United States. Although the fact pattern involved only three 2-person teams dispensing variola via low-tech aerosol sprays in shopping malls in Oklahoma City, Atlanta, and Philadelphia, the scenario quickly spun awry. The simulation players included a number of prominent national leaders—such as former senator Sam Nunn (who played the president), former CIA Director James Woolsey, and former FBI Director William Sessions—qualified to carry out their roles in a realistic, knowledgeable way, but they soon lost control of the evolving catastrophe. In the exercise, the nation's entire stockpile of smallpox vaccine was exhausted by the sixth day; the disease had spread to twenty-five states and fifteen foreign countries; and 2,600 people died, with another 11,000 infected.[51]

Among the sobering lessons learned from Dark Winter were the participants' conclusions that a BW attack upon the United States today "could threaten vital national security interests," with massive civilian casualties, breakdowns in essential institutions, and violations of civil liberties; that "current organizational structures and capabilities are not well suited for the management of a BW attack"; and that "there is no surge capability in the US health care and public health systems." In short, the scenario of a successful terrorist use of a smallpox weapon against the civilian population—even one not aided by the most sophisticated technologies that a determined government might be expected to sponsor—was devastatingly effective.[52]

Just as all participants and observers in Dark Winter were shaken by the seeming impossibility of the task, other role-playing and training events have reinforced the importance of attempting to do better. "Operation TOPOFF," a May 2000 Department of Justice exercise featuring a simulated bioterrorism attack on Denver, was among more than two hundred counterterrorism training exercises funded by the federal government since 1996. Many aim to introduce local emergency crews to the stresses they may encounter in those situations of unique disaster and to practice how officials at all levels of government might collaborate in better response. So far, these experiences seem to raise more questions than they answer about how to best organize the country's BW self-defense capabilities.

Moreover, even those "case studies" largely ignored what turned out to be the 2001 terrorists' weapon of choice: ramming civilian airliners into buildings. No structure could be expected to withstand such an overwhelming onslaught, and biological laboratories—no matter how well secured and how swiftly their ordinary protective precautions are upgraded—are as vulnerable as any other. On the morning of September 11, as the world was reeling from calamities in New York, Arlington, Virginia, and Pennsylvania, the Federal Bureau of Investigation alerted officials that there might be yet another hijacked airplane aloft, perhaps headed toward Atlanta and the headquarters of the Centers for Disease Control and Prevention. While the threat turned out to be empty, CDC officials prudently evacuated the building, save for a security presence to safeguard the laboratory contents.

The fall 2001 tragedies also triggered a paradigm shift in public attitudes toward, and awareness of, bioterrorism, illustrating that a heightened concern over terrorists' diverse ambitions and capabilities was dreadfully overdue. What some have referred to as "the changing face of terrorism" makes the analysis of potential biological weapons use both more complex and essential. Today, there is an array of deviant groups with the potential and inclination for inflicting mass harm, and their capabilities for achieving their desperate aims have mushroomed; even our vocabulary has not kept pace: analysts talk of "super-terrorism," "ultra-terrorism," even "post-modern terrorism." They categorize individuals and groups according to their motivations: political (now almost quaintly old-fashioned), religious, apocalyptic, or ethnic; even criminal Mafia-style organizations with financial goals might find a localized use for biological weapons. And, of course, the division between state-sponsored and independent zealots remains important, although perhaps increasingly fuzzy. We have been stunned by how methodical and disciplined the new groups have become; how focused on ambitious, long-term objectives; and how brazen in manipulating American institutions and cultural traditions in executing their plans.

The national response was to gear up our bioterrorism precautions in several directions, with special attention devoted to the monstrous possibility of a deliberate smallpox attack. First, the administration sought an emergency supplemental appropriation of $1.5 billion to procure and administer a massive expansion of the National Pharmaceutical Stockpile. Featured among the antibiotics and vaccines to be acquired was a $500 million increment to enable the production of up to 300 million doses of smallpox vaccine—enough to cover all Americans. As part of that enterprise, the Department of Health and Human Services has negotiated sped-up delivery of smallpox vaccine under an existing contract with OraVax: instead of producing forty million doses by 2004, the company will provide fifty million doses by the end of 2002. The Food and Drug Administration, for its part, has pledged to accelerate its traditionally time-consuming evaluation of new methods for the production of the vaccine. In addition, the existing vaccine stocks could be diluted to cover more people, and the fortuitous discovery of an unknown inventory of 85 million additional doses greatly eased the strain. The government has no plans, as of yet, to begin mass administration of the vaccine, but as HHS Secretary Tommy G. Thompson expressed the goal, there would be substantial psychological comfort in the promise that "Every man, woman, and child will have a vaccine they can say has their name on it."[53]

In addition, the CDC has now vaccinated against variola some 140 members of elite epidemiologic teams, who might be dispatched at short notice to assist local health workers in responding to a smallpox outbreak. Likewise, the government has augmented its outreach programs to train physicians to recognize smallpox cases, differentiate them from other similar-appearing pox illnesses, and administer the vaccine with skill and speed. The idea of a return to mandatory smallpox vaccination of the American civilian population has also been floated, despite the absence of evidence that any massive smallpox attack is imminent, and despite the dangers that such a precaution would entail for the population at large. Even the World Health Organization has reviewed its long-standing guidelines on smallpox vaccination but ultimately reiterated that the now traditional practice (vaccinating only laboratory workers and others exposed to unusual risks) should be sustained.

The events of September and October 2001 also prompted the Bush administration to reverse its predecessors' course regarding eradication of the smallpox virus samples. In November 2001, the United States announced that it would no longer support the World Health Organization's planned variola destruction, at least until a series of stiff new conditions had been satisfied. These included the development of a new, safer vaccine; the discovery of two independent antiviral medications; the creation of new capabilities for detecting and identifying variola in the environment and in the human body; and even the acquisition of the ability to counteract genetically modified variants of variola. Secretary Thompson declared that in the changed world of bioterrorism, the threat of smallpox demanded greater attention: "Until we have developed our defenses, we must keep this killer secure but available for needed research."[54]

Overall, the national sense of urgency has sometimes teetered on the verge of panic or at least on a profound sense of paralyzing helplessness—it was difficult to conceptualize a response that could adequately cope with the unknown, poorly characterized, and seemingly invisible onslaught of biological terrorism. While the country was earnestly trying to "do more" to gird itself against this novel threat, the apprehension lingered that our shocking vulnerability was due, not exclusively to poor preparation or insufficient attention to the threat, but in disconcertingly large measure to the sheer intractability of the danger itself—would *anything* suffice to rescue us from this horrible scourge?

The case study of Aum Shinrikyo, the millennialist cult that released a small quantity of low-grade sarin nerve gas on the Tokyo subway in April 1995 illustrates those difficulties. In that episode, a wealthy, but not especially coherent, collection of nonexperts assembled the CW wherewithal for killing twelve people, sending 5,000 more to hospitals with a variety of ailments, and terrorizing untold millions in Japan and elsewhere. The sarin used by the group was impure, and the rudimentary packages they placed on the subway trains failed to disperse it optimally; more sophisticated technology would surely have led to a higher death toll. Likewise, if the cult had succeeded in its earlier enterprises involving biological weaponry—members had previously attempted to acquire Ebola virus samples for possible weapons use, and they did accumulate, experiment with, and attempt to deploy, both anthrax and botulism toxin, before reverting to chemical weapons—the outcome may have been a great deal worse. Now that the psychological barrier against that sort of unconventional "superterrorism" has been breached, will other misguided groups and individuals be far behind? And will they not have taken the time to learn from the technical missteps of Shoko Asahara and his deviant band?

Inside the United States, amateur BW terrorists had emerged long before September 11, 2001, to assert their ugly capabilities. The most notorious—some say, the first successful—such attack came in 1984, when disciples of Bhagwan Shree Rajneesh, a commune leader in Oregon, deliberately contaminated a series of local restaurant salad bars with salmonella bacteria. The deranged goal, reportedly, was to sicken, but not kill, townspeople, in order to prevent them from voting in a municipal election that threatened the commune's perquisites. More than 750 people came down with food poisoning (with no fatalities) as a result. The pathogen had been purchased legally from a commercial source, and the commune had built up a substantial covert biological weapons infrastructure.

Other illustrations of BW terrorist threats, hoaxes, or attempts had also begun to accumulate. In 1995, Larry Wayne Harris, a Lancaster, Ohio, microbiologist and neo-Nazi, obtained—by a simple telephone order from a respected supplier—freeze-dried samples of *Yersinia pestis*, the bacterium that causes bubonic plague. His articulated purpose was to develop a vaccine to counteract what he foresaw as an imminent attack of "Iraqi rats carrying supergerms." At that time, it was not illegal to acquire the agent by unverified telephone or mail order (the regulations have since been tightened),[55] but Harris was apprehended for fraud (i.e., falsely representing his credentials and facilities) when the sales staff was tipped off by his overeagerness to receive the pathogen. Three years later, he was arrested again, this time in possession of what he claimed was enough military grade anthrax to "wipe out all of Las Vegas." Experts debate whether Harris truly fits the definition of a "terrorist"— his activities have not yet harmed anyone—but he illustrates the danger a lone sociopath can pose, if equipped with minimal amounts of funding, technological knowledge, persistence, and motivation.[56]

A 1997 incident—of a sort now all too typical—provided an early template illustrating the reaction that BW carries for the public at large, as well as for security and health officials. The national headquarters of the Jewish organization B'nai B'rith in Washington, D.C., received in the ordinary mail a mysterious package labeled *anthrax* and oozing with a red gelatinous substance. The material, and the threat behind it, were quickly identified as bogus, but in the melee, authorities sealed off the building for eight hours, quarantined one hundred people, and hosed down another fourteen people with disinfectant on the public sidewalks. The surrounding neighborhood was a jumble of emergency vehicles for hours, and the psychic cost for the victims of the hoax, and for others, was substantial.

For whatever perverse reason, bioterrorism hoaxes—especially those involving phony claims of an anthrax weapon—proliferated. Bioterrorism expert Jessica Stern tabulated no fewer than forty-seven such incidents in the United States in the mid- to late-1990s, prompting a surge in statutory and regulatory efforts to put more teeth into the law enforcement response and more certainty into the public health capabilities. Other studies, using different definitions of CBW terrorism, have identified hundreds of occasions—of varying intensity and effectiveness—of possible terrorist threat or use of those capabilities in the United States and around the planet.

In this context, the massive wave of anthrax activity in late 2001—a handful of actual cases, a larger grouping of dangerous exposures, and an expanding incidence of threats and hoaxes—should be viewed as the inevitable culmination of the trend. Each isolated case has to be taken seriously; each report of a "mysterious white powdery substance" provokes a full-scale response, often with police and health care workers clad in full body protective "moon suits." The public has become intimately familiar with the previously obscure differences between cutaneous and inhalational anthrax, and the community's apprehensions have intensified. Laboratories and other facilities have sputtered to increase their security precautions, though not sure of the exact threats to guard against. The uncertainty is compounded by not knowing who is responsible—Afghanistan-based terrorists responding to the U.S. military campaign, some homegrown deviants, or a mixture of sources.

Moreover, it is not only anthrax that lies in the terrorists' medicine cabinet. The potential for weaponization of smallpox also plays a role in many of the nation's uncertainties and contradictory considerations. The CDC, on the one hand, reportedly considers smallpox to be a major terrorist threat; the FBI, on the other hand (focusing on the difficulty that nonstate actors would likely experience in attempting to obtain variola samples) does not mention small-pox on its roster of germs of concern.

Variola genuinely belongs on anyone's "short list" of potential military or terrorist vehicles. Some would consider variola the "ideal" BW agent for small armies or for nonstate actors because of the lethality of the virus, the absence of any cure, and the loathing the disease has always inspired. Moreover, small-pox meets many of the BW protagonist's other likely desiderata due to the virus's ability to be produced quickly, its sufficient stability for storage and transportation, its ability to be disseminated in an effective manner, the self-protection the user can undertake through vaccination, and the stress the disease would put on national health care systems. Unlike some other potential BW agents (such as anthrax), smallpox is communicable from one person to another; unlike some others (such as plague) the disease agent is robust, capable of persisting in the environment for a sustained period.

At the same time, there are contraindications regarding variola as a biological weapon: for all its historic damage, smallpox has been reined in by an effective (albeit imperfect) protective vaccine; variola is not the easiest substance to manipulate and to weaponize; it would be very difficult for anyone today to obtain variola stocks without at least the passive cooperation or active collaboration of a government (or a key employee) possessing clandestine or overt stocks; and the disease may be deemed too slow for optimal military or terrorist applications, because of the lag time between an initial exposure and the emergence of incapacitating/lethal conditions (and before the disease can be communicated to other potential victims).

Scientific study of the virus now also affects its weapons potential. Analysts have for some time been committed to exploring the variola DNA structure (preparatory either to eradicating it or to developing better means of counter-acting it). Those efforts have resulted, inter alia, in revealing the complete DNA sequencing of several strains of the virus, and further analysis is under way to map still other varieties in equal detail. Researchers have published the results in scientific journals and on the Internet; as the other contributions are com-pleted, the benefits of this microscopic learning will again be widely shared, to assure everyone that the acquired data are not being hoarded for one-sided military advantage.

However, some observers now contend that such publication could be a tragic error, because it could provide any hostile government or terrorist organization with a blueprint for reconstructing (and perhaps improving) the deadly virus. The notion of stiff voluntary or mandatory restrictions on the dissemination of such data has arisen, with the danger of increased government censorship of dual-use information, and the criticism that biology must "lose its innocence" in order to safeguard the community against a terrorist's applications of basic learning.

In sum, as George Tenet, director of the U.S. Central Intelligence Agency, testified, the threat of unconventional terrorism inside the United States "is real, it is immediate, and it is evolving."[57] After the September 11, 2001, attacks, Attorney General John Ashcroft upped the rhetorical ante, saying "Terrorism is a clear and present danger to Americans today" and noting that at least in the immediate future, the likelihood of deadly attacks may only rise.[58]

BWC PROTOCOL NEGOTIATIONS

In response to these diverse pressures, the world community has once again taken up the diplomatic cudgel, attempting to craft a mutually acceptable augmentation of the Biological Weapons Convention, the primary (although imperfect) bulwark that international law has offered to foreclose biological hostilities. The goal, expressed with different degrees of fervor by different participants, is to formulate new institutions and procedures that will enhance parties' confidence in each other's compliance, through reporting mechanisms, on-site visitation, and strengthened enforcement capabilities.

The halting progress, for more than a decade, toward such a protocol reflects the attempts to balance the arms control interest in greater openness (e.g., to require documentation from, and international inspectors' access into, military and dual-capable facilities) with the continued protection of each country's national security secrets and each laboratory's confidential business information (e.g., to ensure that data that are militarily useful or commercially valuable are safeguarded). It is a most challenging diplomatic balancing act, and it is not surprising that the multilateral wrangling proceeds at a glacial pace. Indeed, given the complexity of the competing interests, and the financial and national security interests at stake, it is perhaps noteworthy that any headway at all has been registered: for many years, the U.S. government resisted convening any such negotiations, on the ground that it would be impossible to craft a mutually tolerable, legally binding instrument that would appropriately pursue both such diametrically opposed desiderata.

In the summer of 2001, just when it appeared that success might finally be within sight, the negotiations were dealt a possibly fatal blow. The Bush administration declared its opposition to the delicate compromises that were then emerging from the bargaining. The United States concluded that the draft protocol was irretrievably defective in two respects: First, it failed to provide a sufficiently vigorous inspection apparatus for deterring and detecting violations. Second, the intrusions it did allow would be unacceptably expensive for industry, compromising industrial secrets in the biotech industry. America would therefore not approve the nascent document, or even support additional negotiations to emend it.

The United States asserted that it was not completely abandoning the effort to develop a more effective BWC and that it would pursue alternative approaches to strengthening the regime in the future. These could include reciprocal commitments for each country to pass domestic legislation outlawing individual citizens' actions in contravention of the treaty; to grant blanket permission for international extradition of any violators; and to improve oversight of high-risk experiments and of access to dangerous microorganisms. The American concepts would also incorporate establishment of a United Nations procedure for investigating suspicious outbreaks of diseases or allegations of BW use, and a voluntary mechanism for clarifying concerns about compliance via exchanges of information or on-site visits. A "code of conduct" to guide future bioethics research could also be developed.

The international community (many of whom had their own doubts about the viability of the draft protocol) then paused, awaiting further clarification of Washington's next move. Many expressed dismay that the fight against bioterrorism might become yet another manifestation of America's unilateralist approach to complicated, shared problems of global concern and that the BWC might suffer irretrievably in the bargain. In December, the United States further validated many of those fears, abruptly proposing to terminate the protocol negotiations altogether, a move that caused the treaty review conference to dissolve in disarray and uncertainty over what would come next in the struggle to erect effective international legal barriers against biological warfare. The process of trying to pick up the pieces of the diplomatic effort—or to determine whether aspects of the new U.S. proposals can help bridge the gap between America and the rest of the BWC parties—resumes in November 2002.

OFFENSIVE AND DEFENSIVE COMPETITION

A final aspect of the military dimension of smallpox elimination involves the curious international offense/defense arms race that each country active in the BW arena is necessarily engaged in. Every effort (or every fear of an enemy's effort) to develop a new type of germ warfare, or to invent an improved type of dispersal mechanism, may elicit diametrically opposing efforts to assist the potential victims. Two relationships emerge from this interaction.

First, the "defensive" side of the ledger is behind in this competition, and may be destined to stay in arrears indefinitely. As noted above, it may always be easier, cheaper, and quicker to develop new offensive biological weapons—genetically engineered viruses, bacteria that can evade existing antibiotics, and so on—than to derive appropriate vaccines and other countermeasures against them. The U.S. military is resisting any defeatism on this score and is pursuing important defensive programs, reacting both to the Iraqi surprises of Desert Storm and to the events of September 11, 2001. Improved sensors are a current top priority, as the Pentagon recognizes the imperative for earlier, more discriminating evaluation of mysterious powders, invisible residues, and oncoming clouds of potentially BW-laden gas. Better protective gear is sought, too, to shield troops, civilians, equipment, and installations. Broadly effective vaccines or multispectrum antiviral medications would be the Holy Grail of the BW defense research effort. Research into improved antivariola vaccines and treatments is, of course, a focus of special interest. But a sense remains that the defenses are perpetually doomed to playing "catch-up," trying urgently to respond to a potential aggressor's hard-to-anticipate next move. Vulnerability to BW and bioterrorism, therefore, may be an inherent feature of modern life.

CARL A. RUDISILL LIBRARY
LENOIR-RHYNE COLLEGE

Second, defensive research and development activities take place under the shadow of dual capability. Wide applicability of knowledge means that improvements in defenses may also automatically enable improvements in offenses, because the knowledge gained on one side of the ledger can so easily be applied to the other. A country that invents a secret new vaccine, for example, may feel more free to use the relevant pathogen in offensive combat, knowing that it has achieved a one-sided margin of safety. Outside observers, accordingly, cannot easily retain confidence that any country's new medications, equipment, and protective capabilities will be pursued solely for peaceful purposes. Any major activity in the BW area, therefore, regardless of its true, benign motivations, will likely instill fear, or at least concern, in other countries, who will worry that ambiguous activities might be distorted, sooner or later, for aggressive ends. As Susan Wright has observed,

Paradoxically, striving for a perfect defense against all conceivable biological warfare agents is not merely futile, but likely actually to foster the discovery of novel biological weapons. And because it is so hard to be sure of the motives behind such programs, other nations are likely to carry out ambiguous and provocative programs of their own. The result could well be a dangerous and destabilizing race to explore the weapons implications of advances in the biological sciences.[59]

CONCLUSION

This examination of the military dimension of the smallpox story provides several cautionary notes. First, military officials around the world and throughout history have always taken accidental outbreaks of smallpox into account as sometimes cataclysmic influences upon the fortunes of war. Moreover, various armies have routinely conceptualized the variola virus as a potential biological warfare agent, and they have occasionally experimented with it and stockpiled it on a "standby" basis—tons of it, in the case of the USSR.

Smallpox is one of the very few biological weapons that has been used in combat: a variety of military officials, employing an array of techniques, have attempted to use the virus deliberately to sow illness among the enemy. Genetic engineering now augurs an ability to alter the variola DNA into an even nastier type of germ, one with even fewer limitations upon its battlefield potential. Proliferation is also a growing concern: more and more countries, it appears, retain at least a latent interest in a BW program, and some of them may have focused on smallpox. And just as distressing, in the early days of the twenty-first century, the apparition of terrorist use of a variola weapon appears even more ominous—many would call smallpox an "ideal" terrorist implement, if the evildoers could just get their hands on the stuff.

There are few instances in human history in which a weapon system was available, and seemed to offer some degree of military advantage, yet was *not* used in combat. The "fog of war" and the political and personal pressures of national combat tend to drive belligerents to exploit any possible security advantage. In an era where the leading legal impediments to the use of smallpox and other biological agents—the 1925 Geneva Protocol and the 1972 Biological Weapons Convention—are widely perceived as incomplete, insufficiently rigorous, and under stress, the maintenance of a BW-free planet seems in jeopardy.

Those considering national security, therefore, speak only equivocally about the concept of variola extermination. On the one hand, it is only by eliminating this pathogen completely that we could be certain that a smallpox weapon would never be wielded against our troops or our civilian population in future international combat or domestic terrorism. Only by strengthening the norm against the whole concept of biological warfare can we reinforce our security in the notion that if hostilities must come, at least they will retain that veneer of civilization. On the other hand, until all corners of the world are safely, and verifiably, rid of all BW—a goal that national sovereignty and concerns for privacy have always impeded and that advances in biotechnology now push still further into the imagination—we cannot be certain that the threat has reliably and permanently been turned off. In that milieu, perhaps a small residue of variola, as a standard against which to compare any emergent "designer bugs," and as a template for focused antiviral research, would still be a prudent safeguard.

CHAPTER 4

ENVIRONMENTAL LAW AND POLICY

Concern over the full panoply of environmental issues—coupled with a (somewhat belated) realization that many significant environmental problems must be conceptualized in global terms—is burgeoning. Although policy-makers, legislators, and litigants have not yet turned their environmental law focus onto the arcane world of the variola virus, they have crafted treaties, statutes, regulations, and other pronouncements that demand our atten-tion—at least for the purpose of considering whether the rhetoric, policy ori-entations, and strategic choices reflected in the growing corpus of domestic and international environmental law can shed light on our current smallpox dilemma.

LEGAL BACKGROUND

Although shards of an ancient environmental law can be discerned throughout history, the modern incarnation—or at least environmental law as a distinct, recognized discipline—dates back only four decades or so in the United States and claims even more recent origins in most other countries. Appreciation for *international* environmental law as a discrete topic of inquiry is even younger;

only with the United Nations' watershed Conference on the Human Environment, convened in Stockholm in 1972, did the world begin to speak as one (and even then, with considerable cacophony) on this set of shared ecological issues.[1]

Once environmentalism gained a small place in the American and global public and legal consciousness, it started a swift ascent that shows little sign of abating. United States statutory regulation of environmental matters certainly displayed early exponential growth: the National Environmental Policy Act (NEPA) of 1969 begat the Clean Air Act of 1970 and the Clean Water Act of 1977; the Marine Mammal Protection Act of 1972 was followed by the Endangered Species Act of 1973; the Toxic Substances Control Act of 1976 led to the Comprehensive Environmental Response Compensation and Liability Act of 1980; and so on.[2]

Likewise, international environmental law caught the zeitgeist of the era. From modest origins, the family of bilateral and multilateral treaties dealing in some large measure with environmental protection or remediation has swollen to nine hundred or more.[3] Some of these (like some of the statutes) are only partial measures, reflecting an incomplete consensus on the nature of the problems and the practicable solutions to them. And some international instruments were never intended to have legally binding force or have yet to attract widespread adherence—including, in several instances, lacking the participation of the United States. But overall, they bespeak a growing appreciation for environmental concerns and a commitment to concerted, emphatic action to address them. A leading 1972 international instrument reflects this judgment, calling environmental protection "the urgent desire of the peoples of the whole world and the duty of all Governments."[4]

None of these legal tools is directly relevant to the novel question of preservation or destruction of the smallpox virus. That microbe is too obscure, and the political, legal, moral, and other questions it presents are too avant garde, to have entered into this milieu of public policy. Still, some bits of environmental practice, both domestic and international, are partially relevant, offering us a rich source of analogies, a fountain of compelling rhetoric, and a suggestion of public strategies and perspectives that help illuminate a path, suggesting that the environmental dimension, like the companion perspectives surveyed in other chapters, requires our analysis.

BIOLOGICAL DIVERSITY AS A CRITICAL PARAMETER

The subfield of environmental concerns within which the questions of variola extermination fit most closely is the niche assigned for protection of wildlife, natural habitats, and biological diversity (or biodiversity). While much of environmental law lends itself to pigeonholing, with families of statutes or treaties devoted to tackling more-or-less discrete issues such as air pollution, water pollution, hazardous wastes, and so on, the problem of biodiversity is more complex and more ephemeral, engaging a diffuse concern for the preservation of the variety of life forms in our planet's marvelous genetic stockpile.

In some ways, it may appear odd that the conservationists' instinct here is not to preserve *lives,* per se, but life *forms,* to retain the number of species (and, secondarily, the range of genetic variation within each species). The challenge is not crudely to maximize the number of creatures—plant and animal, large and small—that the earth supports but to ensure that as much as possible of the heterogeneity continues to be available.

And the current realm of biodiversity is thrilling, to be sure—even if we have hardly begun to appreciate and understand its full breadth. To date, humans have described and cataloged between 1.4 and 1.75 million species, which may account for perhaps 10 percent of the true range of biological variation on the planet (excluding microorganisms).[5] Not surprisingly, the larger and more familiar genres of flora and fauna have been analyzed most completely: we know of 4,000 kinds of mammals, 9,000 birds, 6,300 reptiles, and 4,180 amphibians.[6] But the largest families of living creatures comprise among the smallest and most obscure individuals: there are at least 50,000 species of mollusks, 10,000 ferns, and 69,000 kinds of fungi, and by far the most diverse group of creatures is the insects, with some 750,000 or more known species.[7] We know so little about the smallest creatures that even the experts are simply guessing how many types of bacteria and other microscopic entities the earth may currently bear. And we are discovering and cataloging new species with remarkable frequency: hundreds of new creatures are formally described for the first time each year. Even within the most-studied realms, there are still occasional surprises: an average of two new bird species is discovered each year, and several new mammals, including primates, have been found and cataloged for the first time within the past several years.[8]

This array, of course, is not distributed uniformly across the planet. A small and diminishing number of biodiversity "hot spots" account for a disconcerting percentage of the earth's species: coral reefs, coastal estuaries, and tropical rain forests are the true preserves of biodiversity. And these repositories are under incessant attack: between 1960 and 1990, one-fifth of all tropical rain-forest cover was lost, and the onslaught against the remainder has continued at 1 to 2 percent per year.[9]

This analysis should not suggest that the earth's cadre of biological exemplars could ever be constant. In fact, species come and go with an irregularity and unpredictability that masks a statistical likelihood: the average life span of a species is between one and ten million years. Some last much longer; other "experimental" life forms disappear quickly in failure—"genetic erosion" is thus an inescapable fact of life.

Moreover, even large-scale erasures of species are recurrent events. The fossil record documents five distinct episodes of massive extinctions of species, triggered by climate change, meteor strikes, and so forth, when 50 percent or more of the existing animal species disappeared "suddenly" (when measured by geological time frames). The last of these, at the end of the Cretaceous period, brought the extermination of the dinosaurs, some sixty-five million years ago. But the planet recovered—on the unimaginable time frame of millions of years—through the evolutionary magic of genetic mutation and natural selection. Today, the earth enjoys more different species than at any other single point in its four-billion-year history, although it is also true that 98 percent of the species that have ever lived have long since gone extinct.

We stand now on the precipice of a sixth great wave of species exterminations, an occasion different from the earlier shocks both because it will be the first such transformation caused, or at least materially assisted, by human beings, and also because it is progressing at unprecedented speed. Evolutionary biologists estimate that the earth is now forfeiting 27,000 species per year—seventy per day, one every twenty minutes—roughly 1,000 to 10,000 times the normal "background" rate, and the death march appears to be accelerating.[10] Already, some 24 percent of the various kinds of mammals, 25 percent of fish, 20 percent of reptiles and amphibians, and 11 percent of birds are considered "threatened": either in immediate danger of extinction or vulnerable to extinction. It is altogether possible that we will lose one-quarter to one-half of the life forms on the planet by the middle of this century—a catastrophe eons faster than that which befell the dinosaurs.[11]

Moreover, the decline in the population of a species, even if it is arrested short of total extinction, can itself have cataclysmic effects on biodiversity. As the numbers of individuals remaining in a particular species diminish, their internal genetic variability, the number of distinct strains, and the possibilities for novel recombinations in future generations can be expected to contract, too. The potential for recovery of the species to its original full strength is compromised, as the robustness of the organism's genetic possibilities is diminished and can never be exactly recompensed.

The human contribution to the sixth wave of extinctions is as multifarious as it is unmistakable. Some species have been lost or jeopardized through overhunting or overfishing: when people "harvest" their prey beyond the sustainable level, permanent population loss may ensue. Pollution of all sorts has its consequences, too, as some organisms are not hardy enough to withstand the toxins dumped into their habitats. Introduction of nonnative competitive or predatory species is part of the story, as well, and there have been numerous examples in which humans have deliberately or inadvertently transported exotic fish, land animals, or plants into a new environment, where the introduced species then consume the native species beyond the self-sustaining level or simply overwhelm their capacity to grow and reproduce. And most spectacularly today, the quest for modern development has driven people to dam rivers, drain wetlands, break prairies, and—most prominently at the moment—to torch their rain forests at an incredible pace.

In all those instances, human beings (whether ancient hunter-gatherers or modern real estate tycoons) did not consciously decide to eradicate the victimized species: those losses were largely the unintended, unanticipated consequences of the individual acts of economic self-promotion. But the net result is that extinction, once entirely a "natural" process, occasioned by inexorable environmental forces, has now become in large measure a "social" process, driven by human activity, preferences, and will.

Humans do, of course, sometimes unite to try to protect selected species or even whole segments of the natural environment. International and domestic legal tools have been crafted to promote the interest in large cetaceans (whales, dolphins, etc.), particular classes of fish, and numerous other species. Yet there is a degree of arbitrariness, even irrationality, in the various discrete selections of protected creatures. For example, the most favored animals are sometimes, but not always, those with the greatest identifiable economic value. They are frequently the large, well-known "charismatic megafauna" that people have the greatest affinity for, fear of, or ability to identify with. And there is often a disconnection between our general interest in preserving a species and our ability to fashion a systematic plan for doing so, or our willingness to pay the price, in economic development or other human enterprises, necessary to validate our abstract concerns.

The consequences of this ongoing free fall in global biodiversity may be difficult to pinpoint but are surely substantial. One category of problems, surveyed in chapter 6, concerns the ethics of species eradication, asking how it can be considered just or proper, for human beings—just one species out of millions on the planet—to exploit, devastate, and waste the genetic potential of so many others.

The other set of reasons "why biodiversity matters" arises from the value of species variation—the economic and other consequences for humans of squandering the inherited range of earthly creation (including the enormous diversity among microorganisms, including viruses). Two subcategories of arguments can be constructed: those having greater application and those having lesser application to the peculiar circumstances of the variola virus.

First, the general proposition for preservation of diversity begins with the observation of the intricate, unfathomable role that the multiplicity of species performs in nature. Most obviously, humans depend upon a wide array of plants, animals, bacteria, fungi, and other life forms for a cornucopia of products: foodstuffs, fuel, drugs, chemicals, fibers, construction materials, and so much more. Just as important is the array of services: photosynthesis, water purification, climate stabilization, flood control, pollination, decomposition, and disposal of wastes, to name just a few. All of these are essential to our life processes, they require multiple sources and agents, and they depend on a delicate interaction between diverse, often unseen, biological agents, large and small. Any calculation of the value of these diverse "ecological goods and services" must remain largely abstract, grounded on the facts that they could not be performed on the requisite scale in any other fashion and that without them human beings could not long survive on the planet. Even with those caveats, one bold calculation estimates their worth at $16–54 trillion per year.[12]

More narrowly, the breadth of life forms seems to be valuable for sustaining natural processes themselves. That is, a diverse environmental community, consisting of a large variety of types of plants and animals, appears to be more stable, more adaptable to perturbations, and less susceptible to disruption from exogenous invaders. A "healthy" and diverse ecosystem, in this sense, is one in which many of the available niches are exploited by divergent species, so while incremental changes will accrete over time, sudden wide-scale losses are less likely.

Finally, appropriate diversity enables us to avoid "putting all our eggs into one basket," by ensuring a multiplicity of resources. If a specific type of onslaught occurs—a new disease, for example, or a sustained change in temperature or hydrology—then, while some species (or groups of species) may suffer, the odds are better that there will be markedly different creatures who can survive or even thrive. The greater the variability in the stockpile, the greater are the chances of withstanding the disruption. In contrast, the increasing reliance that modern agriculture has placed on a small number of highly specialized crops and herds runs a substantial risk: as long as conditions are favorable, the single "best" strain of corn, rice, sheep, or cattle can produce the maximal yields, but if a novel fungus, pest, or disease strikes, the practice of monoculture can result in sudden, catastrophic losses.

The power of the above arguments, however compelling in the general or "ordinary" case of biodiversity, is mostly lost on variola. That virus does not perform valuable environmental services for humankind or the planet. It does not contribute to environmental stability or assist in warding off interlopers. Whether we focus on the pre-1970s environment, when variola was "at large," endemic in much of the world, or on the period since the World Health Organization's successful campaign to reduce the virus to an artificial "range" confined to test tubes in two freezer units, there is little genuine ecological utility realized from variola today.

Therefore, the chief contribution that an awareness of biodiversity can make to our understanding of the smallpox question must lie in the second subargument, the appreciation for the hypothetical: who knows what uses we might find in the future for this tidbit of viral genetic material? The world of environmental biology, after all, is characterized by "unknown unknowns"—that is, at the present time, we don't even know what kinds of things we don't know, and our ability to predict future needs, dangers, and opportunities is sharply circumscribed. Human experience has repeatedly demonstrated that a great many wild species, resources, and wilderness areas were formerly dismissed as worthless and "wastage," but more recent innovations and increased scientific understanding have opened our eyes to their incalculable value and irreplaceable role in essential ecosystems. Once the virus is destroyed, however, any potential service it might one day render is lost forever.

We do know that wild species have always represented a trove of value for people and that we have far from exhausted their potential. One often cited example: of the top 150 prescription drugs in use in the United States, 118 are based on natural sources—74 percent of those are drawn from plants, 18 percent from fungi, 5 percent from bacteria, and 3 percent from vertebrates.[13] Genetic manipulation techniques will surely expand this pattern. Another example: genetic infusions from wild species of grains have repeatedly proven critical in rescuing us from our narrow focus on specific crop species when sudden adverse conditions threaten a catastrophe. In this vein, sometimes the smallest, most noxious, and dangerous pests have turned out to contain significant value, discovered through serendipity or intense research.

In short, the "cautious" argument for preserving biodiversity, even in situations where the potential benefit of retaining a particular species looks so thin, is that we can never know what utility our successors might find in an organism we disrespect today. At a time when such a high percentage of the available species has not been studied or even discerned, there are millions of what William H. Rogers Jr. calls "unread books."[14] How can we discard any one of them, even if a glance at its cover suggests only a story of agonizing disease and suffering?

The literature, as well as the law, of environmental protection reflects an unswerving support for the concept of biodiversity and substantial alarm at the current, accelerating rate of its loss. Still, despite all that sensitivity to genetic resources, a virus, and the variola virus in particular, represents something of the limiting case of humanity's proper concern for species preservation. First, this is just one species, out of hundreds or thousands that are now disappearing.

Even the most ardent proponents of biodiversity focus on the "big picture," the mass accumulation or detraction of genetic resources of global proportions. The peril of any one kind of creature, even one as notorious and unique as variola— and even one where the eradication would be deliberate, rather than a by-product of human inattention or neglect—hardly tips the scales of this rich planet.

Second, this particular life form has already been removed from nature, and no one's concept of the pristine environment or respect for biodiversity would entail a deliberate return of the virus to its original, "natural" place in the world, replete with its deadly infection of human beings. So whatever the preservation, use, or potential use of the virus might be, it would have to occur in vitro, or under the most tightly controlled experimental regimes. This is not at all akin to preserving endangered gray wolves for reintroduction into Yellowstone National Park or to salvaging the remnants of an aquatic plant that might one day be able to recapture its former natural range in the Chesapeake Bay once unwanted competitors are checked. We have already irretrievably tinkered with the natural order of things by excluding variola from the human environment, and whatever means we may now select to preserve its DNA chains, they will not resume their prior, or any other, viable ecological niche.

Third, there may be little human "utility" left in variola, other than helping us to concoct better defenses against itself. As noted in chapter 2, underway or contemplated laboratory research might lead to the synthesis of improved antiviral medications or vaccines, targeted against the threat of smallpox as a biological weapon or terrorist device. And it is possible, more generically, that investigation of the unique properties of this highly specialized virus may provide better understanding of the human immune system applicable to other diseases. But it is hard to assess the likelihood of those breakthroughs, the timetable on which they may occur, the costs and benefits of their development, and the opportunity cost of foregone research on other, perhaps even more promising, rare organisms.

Finally, the case of variola is legally and factually anomalous because of its odd configuration of financial incentives, unrepresentative of the usual controversy over protecting an endangered species. That is, the virus presents no conundrum about the limits of sustainable development—the usual staple of this field—where humans have to ponder how fully they can exploit a particular biological resource without choking off its natural replenishment. There is no hunting or fishing of variola; nor does protection of its critical habitat inhibit the construction of new highways or the logging of virgin forests. So just as there is seemingly little to be gained from preserving this species (or, at least, perhaps less to be gained than might be expected from retention of other novel, useful, not-fully-known species), there is little cost in doing so (or, at least, less cost than arises in some other instances of competition over incompatible land uses).

At this juncture in the analysis, many environmental advocates would urge application of the "precautionary principle," inserting a thumb on the scale on the side of human self-restraint. If we do not fully understand what is at stake in a particular environmental issue, if we cannot discern with confidence the pluses and minuses of proceeding with a proposed course of action, we should "play it safe," avoiding irreversible consequences. The absence of definitive proof about hazards, they say, should not be taken as proof of their absence, and the burden should be placed on proponents of an action to demonstrate the safety of departing from the status quo.

Even if one adopts that precautionary mode, however, its application to the current question is problematic. Which course of action is truly "safer" here? Should we prudently avoid irreversible outcomes by preserving the virus, at least for now? Or should we cautiously seek to minimize the social dangers by destroying the last variola stockpiles as soon as possible, in order to eliminate the specter that smallpox could somehow leak out, once again inflicting its horrors upon humanity? If we do retain the virus, do we allow research with it, to develop better tools to combat smallpox, or do we permanently lock the freezer doors, to guard against disastrous accidents? The precautionary principle offers scant guidance on weighing such incommensurate risks; even if people everywhere were committed by consensus to a cautious approach, how would we interpret that mandate here?

Sophisticated environmental law, both international and domestic, is all about risk. We try to evaluate the range of likely dangers, assess their respective probabilities and costs, and construct pathways (which usually carry their own set of costs and dangers) to minimize or mitigate them. Unfortunately, we can rarely achieve a zero level of risk—at least not in the most interesting, important, and controversial cases. Viewed in this way, variola seems to offer us a unique opportunity: to remove a harmful substance entirely from the environment. Or does it? Does the specter of hidden virus stockpiles somewhere on the planet relegate the smallpox issue to a more familiar, but equally ineffable, calculus: Can we evaluate the risks of continued retention versus the asymmetric risks of destruction? And the possibility of *benefits* from retention—for example, experiments to develop improved vaccines or to better understand human organ "rejection" phenomena—makes the choice even harder.

Comparative risk analysis is a young field in environmental law and elsewhere. Even in traditional environmental settings, experts dispute the methodologies of cost/benefit analysis that seek to monetize the discounted present value of gains and losses. In this novel area of decision making, the absence of a coherent framework of analysis is not surprising—we are essentially at the limits of society's ability to make rational choices.

In general, environmentalists stress the preferred approach of serving biodiversity by maintaining species in their natural settings, with all the attendant "connections" to other species that occur in the wild. This bias in favor of *in situ* preservation reflects the appreciation that the full functioning of a living being cannot be divorced from its interactions with its surroundings; any isolation, removal, or resiting carries an element of artificiality, and to truly understand and protect a species, we should sustain it in a "normal" habitat.

Sometimes, however, that preferred option is unobtainable, either because of destruction of the species' natural milieu for other human uses or, as in the case of variola, because of the inherent, unavoidable danger of the creature itself. International law, science, and policy thus recognize the subsidiary value of *ex situ* preservation, in nature preserves, zoos, and other institutions where the species can be safely sustained. Laboratories, gene banks, museums, or other depositories for frozen, dried, or other types of specimens are another option, especially promising for seeds, germ plasm, or other genetic materials. Microorganisms, too, can be retained in appropriate "DNA banks," although to date insufficient attention has been paid to this forum for biodiversity.

For the most part, international law insistently favors the natural settings for species, and the documents refer to reserves as only a second-best option (and even in that fallback mode, international law generally advocates locating those artificial reservoirs inside the country of natural origin of the species). But in the case of variola, the most artificial of *ex situ* environments is the only realistically available alternative: it is either preservation via isolation in

American and Russian frozen test tubes (or a modest variation thereupon) or complete eradication. And since every country is a country of origin of variola (although only specific countries have contributed the particular samples now held in the two laboratories), the location of continued storage should not matter very much.

INTERNATIONAL ENVIRONMENTAL LAW

From the most modest (and recent) of origins, there is now a plethora of international legal materials populating the global environmental scene, including hundreds of international agreements and scores more of resolutions from the UN General Assembly and other prestigious multilateral forums. Principles of customary international law likewise are emerging with increased vigor, binding even on countries that have absented themselves from particular environmental treaty obligations.

All of this, it should be noted, has proceeded in a largely ad hoc fashion, lacking centralized oversight or grand strategy, and the result is a patchwork of law imperfectly governing international environmental matters. There are far too many instruments to be surveyed adequately here, but two prominent treaties, as well as several emerging customary and "soft law" commitments and principles must be highlighted for possible relevance to the variola story.

The most salient landmark in this field is the Convention on Biological Diversity, signed at the UN Conference on Environment and Development (the Earth Summit) in Rio de Janeiro in June 1992. Designed as a broad framework instrument, the convention embraces fundamental principles concerning conservation of species, sustainable development of natural resources, and biotechnology. It operates at an abstract and general level, establishing overarching international commitments (often stated with the caveat that parties are obligated to undertake the conservation measures only "as far as possible and as appropriate").[15] These standards are to be supplemented in the years to come by more specific protocols, that is, more detailed commitments containing the "teeth" of the arrangement.

The convention's preamble describes the contracting parties as "Conscious of the intrinsic value of biological diversity and of the ecological, genetic, social, economic, scientific, educational, cultural, recreational, and aesthetic values of biological diversity and its components."[16] It establishes a regime of "common but differentiated responsibilities," under which all states have obligations (including obligations *ergo omnes*—i.e., running to all other states, regardless of where any particular consequences of their actions might happen to fall) to husband genetic resources. But because the various states differ regarding possession of rare species, endangered habitats, wealth, and technology, their specific duties (mostly to be elaborated in the subsequent instruments) will vary.

The Biodiversity Convention has been joined by a remarkable 182 countries, marking its sudden emergence as a lodestar environmental instrument. But the United States remains outside the regime: the first Bush administration declined to sign the treaty (becoming the only industrialized country to hold out at Rio), citing dissatisfaction with several financial aspects. In 1993, the Clinton administration did sign, but the U.S. Senate has to date declined to provide its advice and consent, so the United States stands in considerable isolation in its absence from this key document.

As part of the bargaining between the economically developed countries (often termed "the North") and the still-developing countries ("the South"), the convention addresses—in a compromise, or "fudged" fashion—the allocation of responsibilities for sustaining and exploiting planetary resources. Notably, the negotiators did not label biodiversity as the "common heritage of mankind," a term that had acquired in other United Nations contexts a connotation of international ownership or collective control. Instead, in a rather intricate formula, biological *diversity* is held to be a "common concern" of humankind, while biological *resources* remain the subject of "sovereign rights" of individual states.

These verbal gymnastics mean that each individual country retains unilateral control over its own genetic inheritance, empowered to make national decisions regarding exploitation and protection, while international law contributes the general obligations to conserve biodiversity, to use biological resources in a sustainable manner, and to refrain from causing environmental damage to other states or to global common areas. The general scheme contemplates that the South will allow reasonable access to its genetic resources (e.g., rare plants that could be mined for new pharmaceuticals) and protect them from overdevelopment (e.g., the vanishing rain forests), while the North will provide financial support (e.g., debt forgiveness and "new and additional financial resources"),[17] concessional access to technology, and the benefits of scientific cooperation and advancement. The specifics of any such collaboration—which would establish the Biodiversity Convention as being more than empty rhetoric—are to be developed in the subsequent protocols.

The increasing alarm with which the North has come to view the rampant slash-and-burn pillaging of the tropical rain forests has elicited from the South complaints about hypocrisy: if it was acceptable, perhaps even necessary, for the first states to achieve modern economic development to do so through large-scale manipulation, change, and exploitation of their natural environment, why should the latecomers to technological advancement be any more inhibited? And if the Northern states now suddenly want to preserve more of the earth in its pristine, natural condition, shouldn't they be prepared to share with the desperately poor peoples of the South the financial benefits they have already reaped from altering their own national environmental heritage?

Furthermore, the developed world's newfound conservation instincts ring hollow when the industrialized countries continue to pinch what remains of their own biodiversity reserves. Each time a species is endangered or a natural habitat compromised in the United States, Europe, or other Northern regions, the Southern interlocutors question anew whether the fervent desire to protect the equatorial rain forests is not at least partially a cloak for advanced capitalism's interest in sustaining the underdeveloped regions as weak economies and sources for exploitation, rather than as strong and growing competitors.

Notably, the Biodiversity Convention operates partially on the "micro" level: it defines the protected biological resources as including genetic resources, which, in turn, include genetic material, defined as "any material of plant, animal, microbial or other origin containing functional units of heredity."[18] Even the variola virus, it would seem, would fall within this purview. Most of the operational language of the convention, however, is poised at a more "macro" level, obligating states to "develop national strategies, plans or programmes for the conservation and sustainable use of biological diversity,"[19] without specifying what would be required with respect to any particular plant, animal, or microbe that happens to get in the way of economic "progress."

Finally, the Biodiversity Convention is noteworthy in this context for what it says about the *location* of preservation operations. The parties' expressed preference, reflecting the general orientation noted above, is for local, *in situ* conservation, in natural habitats and natural surroundings. *Ex situ* sanctuaries and reserves are accepted as having an important, usually subsidiary, role to play, which the treaty notes should be "preferably in the country of origin" of the protected species.[20] Again, however, the only acceptable environment for variola now is sterile laboratories, and the "countries of origin" of the samples currently housed in Atlanta and Koltsovo have never requested their repatriation.

In addition to the 1992 global convention signed in Rio, concerned countries have fashioned a series of regional biodiversity conventions, applicable to their respective "neighborhoods," as well as a host of treaties aimed at protecting particular threatened species. Notable among these are the 1940 Convention on Nature Protection and Wildlife Preservation in the Western Hemisphere (the "Western Convention") and the 1968 African Convention on the Conservation of Nature and Natural Resources.

The Western Convention speaks broadly of the American republics' "wishing to protect and preserve in their natural habitat representatives of all species and genera of their native flora and fauna."[21] It calls upon parties to explore establishing national parks and wilderness areas, to regulate the import and export of threatened plants and animals, and to protect endangered species (listed in an annex to the convention) as a matter of "special urgency and importance" and to do so "as completely as possible."[22] The African Convention has similarly ambitious goals of "conservation, utilization, and development" of soil, water, flora, and faunal resources, which "constitute a capital of vital importance to mankind."[23] The African Convention's annex lists two classes of protected species that include scores of mammals, birds, reptiles, amphibians, fish, and plants (but no microscopic entities). The treaty also provides that the convention shall not affect a state's responsibilities for, inter alia, "defence of human life."[24]

The 1973 Convention on International Trade in Endangered Species (widely known as CITES) is the most important, if not always successful, document in this part of the field. It is designed to promote biodiversity by undercutting international commercial opportunities for exploitation of endangered species and by fostering national legislation aimed at choking off the black market in rare (living or dead) plants, animals, their body parts, and products derived from them. The treaty functions as a sort of "border guard," interdicting international traffic that jeopardizes the survival of items listed on three annexes that rank species in varying degrees of jeopardy. It responds to the fact that such trade "is responsible for an estimated 40% of vertebrate species facing extinction."[25]

Now adhered to by 154 states, CITES encompasses some 34,000 animal and plant varieties. Careful not to infringe upon the national perquisites of sovereigns, the treaty records that "peoples and States are and should be the best protectors of their own wild fauna and flora."[26] It does not require any *internal* measures—CITES does not address requirements for national preserves, sustainable development, or pollution control—but instead concentrates on the strategy of "following the money," by scrutinizing international trade.

The appendixes list the species to be protected, including mammals, birds, amphibians, reptiles, fish, mollusks, and one insect (the Mountain Apollo butterfly) but no microscopic creatures and certainly not the variola virus. The definition section implies that covered specimens will be either plants or animals, but that restriction is not quite explicit.

The procedures for adding items to the lists, or for moving species up or down the roster of endangerment, were deliberately kept flexible to allow quick additions in response to changing circumstances; the minimum level of protection can be triggered by any one country unilaterally, not even requiring an affirmative vote from the other parties.

The Convention does not absolutely forbid all trade in the covered items. If the affected states' Scientific Authority and Management Authority (bodies to be designated by each party to implement the purposes of CITES) certify that the specimen was not taken in violation of domestic law and that the trade "will not be detrimental to the survival of that species," it may be licensed for export and import.[27] There is also an exception for scientific research exchanges, allowing the transport for "noncommercial loan, donation or exchange between scientists or scientific institutions . . . of herbarium specimens, other preserved, dried or embedded museum specimens, and live plant material."[28] International traffic in variola specimens, should that ever be undertaken for research purposes, could fit that definition.

Besides the express, legally binding mandates of these and other treaties, the corpus of international environmental law includes two related types of standards that may provide further context for the variola decision. The first, *customary international law,* consists of principles of such widespread acceptance and legitimacy that they are deemed binding upon all countries, even those that have opted out of any applicable treaty. It constitutes a sort of common law of the international system, in which the legal standards are derived from study of what states have done in the real world—what restrictions they consent to implicitly, via their consistent behavior, instead of explicitly via signature on a treaty. The other, related source is often termed *soft law* and incorporates international assertions and declarations that can be quite explicit and vigorous but are not cast in legally binding form or have not yet achieved sufficiently broad acceptance to be compulsory. The dividing line between these two categories is inexact—at what point has a principle of international environmental practice been elevated into the binding category?—and they will be briefly surveyed here in tandem, along with an overview of some of the documents that recognize (or create) them.

The criteria for customary international law can be difficult to state with precision: to rise to this mandatory level, there must be widespread, long-standing concordant state behavior (which can include what a state says, what it does, and what it refrains from saying or doing), motivated by a sense of legal obligation and marked by the acceptance of others. In the environmental field, as elsewhere, this ambiguity permits different understandings about which putative principles have already achieved that status, which are almost there, and which may be beginning to move in that direction.

A most clear-cut illustration of a binding principle of customary international environmental law would be the obligation upon each state to refrain from actions that damage the environment of another country (or the environment of the area outside any country's national jurisdiction—the "global commons," such as Antarctica or the high seas). This rule would be the application to environmental practice of the general international law proposition that countries may not inflict unwarranted harms upon each other—if a state fails to preclude its territory from being used to the serious detriment of another state's air, water, or other resources, it is liable to the innocent victim. Such a mandate of "state responsibility" for its adverse actions has long been reflected in international litigation, in the authoritative *Restatement of the*

Foreign Relations Law of the United States, and in the 1972 Stockholm Declaration of the UN Conference on the Human Environment.

The subsidiary question is whether this obligation to avoid harming the environment of another state has matured into a more generalized obligation to avoid harming the environment per se, regardless of whether the activity in question has evoked the objection of another territorial sovereign. That is, does international law currently have anything to say about a state's *internal* environmental practices; do international standards intrude into *domestic* biodiversity activities?

Some bold international instruments would affirm that they do. The 1972 Stockholm Declaration bluntly asserts that man "bears a solemn responsibility to protect and improve the environment"; that natural resources "must be safeguarded for the benefit of present and future generations"; that earth's capacity to produce resources "must be maintained and, wherever practicable, restored or improved"; and that "Man has a special responsibility to safeguard and wisely manage the heritage of wildlife and its habitat"—all without geographic limitation and without reference to any requirement for particularly aggrieved or victimized states to launch an initial complaint.[29]

Likewise, the "public trust doctrine" would suggest that humans and governments everywhere bear a collective responsibility for safeguarding nature anywhere, that we share a duty to nurture earth's ecological processes, habitats, and populations globally, independent of existing property rights and political boundaries. Temporal as well as geographic borders should not constrain this duty: both the Stockholm and the Rio Declarations speak to the commitment to serve the environmental needs of both present and future generations.

This stewardship duty for nature and natural processes is not confined to selected species in favored, familiar biological niches. One leading "soft law" articulation, the World Charter for Nature—a declaration passed overwhelmingly by the United Nations General Assembly in 1982 (albeit over the dissent of the United States)—contains the most strident expression of a broad duty to all creatures: "Every form of life is unique, warranting respect regardless of its worth to man, and to accord other organisms such recognition, man must be guided by a moral code of action" and "The genetic viability on the earth shall not be compromised; the population levels of all life forms, wild and

domesticated, must be at least sufficient for their survival, and to this end necessary habitats shall be safeguarded." Likewise, it demands, "Natural resources
shall not be wasted, but used with a restraint appropriate to the principles set
forth in the present Charter."[30]

Similarly, the Helsinki "Final Act," a non–legally binding yet authoritative
declaration of the 1975 Conference on Security and Co-operation in Europe,
asserts that the participating nations (including the United States) agree to
cooperate on "Protection of nature and nature reserves; conservation and
maintenance of existing genetic resources, especially rare animal and plant
species."[31]

Not surprisingly, international law contains a partial counterpoint to all that
rhetoric and assertion of common duties. Foremost among these is the
entrenched principle of state sovereignty, which lies at the core of the modern
international system generally and is repeatedly insinuated into international
environmental law in particular.

First, a long line of UN General Assembly resolutions has affirmed, in
varying vocabulary, that each state retains "permanent sovereignty over natural resources," a catchphrase of imprecise meaning but one that asserts the principle that each sovereign, within its national territory, has near plenary authority to address environmental issues including the exploitation, conservation,
and development of its genetic and other resources. The Stockholm Declaration follows suit, averring that "States have, in accordance with the Charter of
the United Nations and the principles of international law, the sovereign right
to exploit their own resources pursuant to their own environmental policies,
and the responsibility to ensure that activities within their jurisdiction or control do not cause damage to the environment of other States or of areas
beyond the limits of national jurisdiction."[32]

The 1992 Rio Declaration, mindful of the poverty-stricken countries' need
for economic advancement, reemphasizes the Stockholm point about states'
"sovereign right to exploit their own resources pursuant to their own environmental and developmental policies," and underscores the importance of "sustainable development."[33]

None of this, of course, was drafted or negotiated with the fate of a tiny virus
in mind. Still, there are hints, suggestions of a global attitude, that provide illu-
mination for our inquiry. The Stockholm Declaration preamble, for example,

contains the straightforward assertion "Of all things in the world, people are the most precious."[34] And common to any notion of generally accepted international law principles would be a right of "survival" or "self-defense"—most frequently asserted in the context of national struggles against foreign aggression but perhaps applicable as well to collective human struggles against other types of alien invaders.

Other emerging principles of customary or soft international law include the obligation to attempt to develop peaceful, consensual, democratic, and scientific solutions to shared environmental problems and to inform, warn, and consult neighboring states before undertaking activities that could carry adverse environmental consequences for them. The Stockholm and Rio Declarations speak to the value of a cooperative spirit and international consensus in reaching decisions on environmental matters, with states participating in collective efforts on an equal footing. Moreover, states are urged to facilitate public awareness of and participation in these decisions, and the value of rational, scientific analysis and planning are stressed, with states encouraged to adopt an integrated and coordinated approach to their developmental planning. Careful and structured analysis of environmental impacts of major actions is explicitly called for: "Environmental impact assessment, as a national instrument, shall be undertaken for proposed activities that are likely to have a significant adverse impact on the environment and are subject to a decision of a competent national authority."[35]

Finally, it is important, for the sake of context, to locate the environmental issues surveyed above within the spectrum of the vast number of international agreements and related instruments protecting selected species, habitats, or environmental processes. Foremost among these would be the 1982 Law of the Sea Convention, widely accepted as "the constitution for the oceans" and dealing with sea-related issues from jurisdiction to exploitation of nonliving resources to deep water fishing. It also supports a dense network of global and regional obligations regarding preservation of the marine environment, and it extends the prior protection of selected "special areas" of the planet, that had been initiated in predecessor instruments applicable to Antarctica, the seabed, and outer space.

Similarly, there is now a library full of other treaties regarding protection of the marine environment (some dealing with particular regions or particular sources of pollution), conservation of biological resources (e.g., selected species of fauna or unusually sensitive areas), cooperation against air pollution or atmospheric degradation, restrictions on the use of toxic chemicals and waste disposal, and many others.

Again, none of these instruments deals with, governs, or explicitly contemplates questions such as the survival or destruction of the remaining samples of the variola virus; they were designed to address issues, regions, and species of quite different characteristics. But some of the vocabulary—the World Charter for Nature's call for respect for "every form of life," for example—rings across the disciplines. When the Biodiversity Convention defines "genetic material" as including "any material of plant, animal, microbial or other origin containing functional units of heredity,"[36] it stretches—perhaps beyond the intention or understanding of its creators—into the world of a virus. Likewise, "Agenda 21," the clarion call from the 1992 Rio de Janeiro Earth Summit, is comparably broad in asserting that "Urgent and decisive action is needed to conserve and maintain genes, species, and ecosystems."[37]

The sentiments of the Rio Declaration that "the precautionary approach shall be widely applied by States"[38] also extend beyond the specific sectors originally at issue. And when the humbling Stockholm observation that "Man is both creature and moulder of his environment"[39] is applied to novel issues, it demands hesitation before any final, irreversible steps are undertaken.

U.S. ENVIRONMENTAL LAW

Turning now from the tools and tactics of international environmental law, we examine next two of the seminal statutes of the United States, one of the leading articulators of domestic environmental protection provisions. Again, any such partial analysis is somewhat misleading—internal American and other national environmental law should be displayed with greater comprehensiveness and subtlety than the current chapter allows—but a brief overview highlights some of the most critical and relevant (or nearly relevant) applications.

The starting point, without doubt, is the National Environmental Policy Act (NEPA) of 1969. The main function of NEPA is procedural: to enforce a requirement for prudent planning, consideration of the full range of environmental issues, and careful evaluation of the feasible alternatives but not to require any particular substantive outcome of that enhanced planning process. That is, after a government agency has thoroughly studied and presented the environmental consequences of its proposed action, and has sincerely assessed the possibilities for remediation of them, it is still empowered to select its favored course of action without environmental constraint, even if it decides to pursue a path that involves considerable pollution, habitat destruction, and waste. The political process (and other, substantive environmental statutes) take over at that point, once NEPA has succeeded in identifying and publicizing the occasion and the circumstances of choice.

More broadly NEPA serves the heuristic function of elevating environmental issues within the consciousness of the bureaucracy, the courts, and the public at large. The purpose of the statute is stated as "it is the continuing policy of the Federal Government . . . to use all practicable means and measures . . . to create and maintain conditions under which man and nature can exist in productive harmony, and fulfill the social, economic, and other requirements of present and future generations of Americans." Both in rhetoric and in effect, NEPA aims to "encourage productive and enjoyable harmony between man and his environment," and to "promote efforts which will prevent or eliminate damage to the environment and biosphere."[40] The National Environmental Policy Act also contains language highlighting the value of preserving an environment that "supports diversity," a notion that was only dimly recognized at the time of the statute's enactment but that has provided a rich basis for subsequent judicial and scholarly commentary.[41]

The statute has subsequently inspired legions of "copycat" enactments among various U.S. states and in many foreign countries. Its ethos has also been extended, mutatis mutandis, to the international arena, where federal agencies are required to recognize the worldwide and long-range character of environmental problems. Moreover, Executive Order 12114, signed by President Carter in 1979, mandates that a similar sort of deliberative assessment is to be undertaken prior to U.S. government activities that may carry significant impacts for the environment outside American jurisdiction.

The teeth of the statute, the well-known requirement for careful, detailed, wide-ranging environmental impact analysis, obliges each agency of the national government to "utilize a systematic, interdisciplinary approach which will insure the integrated use of the natural and social sciences and the environmental design arts in planning and in decisionmaking." The effort is to mandate a rational calculation, with an interdisciplinary "hard science" approach to environmental decisions that were too often previously undertaken in a casual, impressionistic fashion. The law compels the agency to use the environmental impact statement (EIS) process to take a "hard look" at the effects of its proposed action and promote opportunities for the general public to understand and to participate in the process.

So what, if anything, might NEPA require in the case of variola? To date, no federal agencies have accepted the burden of applying the statutory procedures to this issue. Should they? How big a burden (and how big a benefit) would conformity to the statute entail here?

The first of several sequential questions in applying NEPA to the pending destruction of the variola residues is whether the issue involves a proposal for a "major federal action significantly affecting the quality of the human environment." Any activity regarding the virus would be "federal" in character—the Centers for Disease Control, a unit of the U.S. Department of Health and Human Services, is the entity that currently houses, and would eventually be called upon to incinerate, the viral samples, pursuant to World Health Organization determinations. But would the employment of the CDC autoclave here count as "major," with "significant" impact on the environment?

Those key terms defining the scope of NEPA's activities have never been thoroughly plumbed, despite legions of regulatory and judicial attempts to do so. Their application to variola would be even more uncertain. Usually, a "major" action is one involving substantial expenditure of time, money, or other resources—conspicuous, expensive, long-term construction projects are the paradigm here, rather than an activity that could be quickly and cheaply accomplished by a small number of people inside an enclosed laboratory. On the other hand, "major" also means "more than merely routine," which does seem to apply to an unprecedented undertaking that has been years in the making. The statute, moreover, refers to "any irreversible and irretrievable commitments of resources which would be involved in the proposed action should it be implemented."[42] If the variola virus were considered such a "resource," the whole point would be to irreversibly and irretrievably commit it.

Regulations promulgated by the Council on Environmental Quality (CEQ), the federal government's flagship entity for NEPA implementation, identify ten factors for judging the "intensity" of a proposed project, which is key to a finding about its significance. Unfortunately, in this case the different items on that list point in opposite directions. On the one hand, the CEQ suggests that any unique characteristics of the geography of the activity's site should make a difference in assessing its significance—irrelevant here, as is whether the activity would impact items listed in the National Register of Historic Places or violate other federal, state, or local laws.

On the other hand, some factors used by the CEQ to assess intensity have relevance to the variola decision, however it may come out. They include consideration of whether the effects on the quality of the human environment are "highly controversial"; whether those effects "are highly uncertain or involve unique or unknown risks"; whether the action will "establish a precedent" for future iterations; whether the immediate action, even if "insignificant" on its own, is sufficiently related to later proposals that may cumulatively rise to the level of demanding an EIS; and whether the proposed action "affects public health or safety." The possibility of an impact upon any species or habitat determined to be critical under the Endangered Species Act is another relevant criterion, to be discussed further in this chapter. Even "beneficial" effects (e.g., ridding the world of the danger of a smallpox outbreak) can be "significant," prompting the sponsoring agency to prepare an analysis.

It is noteworthy that NEPA places a principal focus on those proposed activities that carry a potential direct impact on the "human environment." The statute and implementing regulations seem to focus primary attention upon consequences for the physical environment, but they also address the wider array of effects that would be experienced principally or exclusively within what is called the social or economic environments. In a nutshell, CEQ regulations and the accompanying case law have more or less resolved this conundrum by concluding that to trigger NEPA processes at all, there must be at least a sufficient impact on the physical environment (so activities that are major only in their effects on social, economic, or other sectors are excluded from coverage), but once that minimal level of physical impact has been reached, the resulting study and documentation are required to delve into the full array of consequences, including the social and economic.

Although there is no statutory "national security" or other generic exception to NEPA that would be relevant here, the EIS and associated requirements can be rendered inapplicable by some other source of law (a subsequent, inconsistent statute or treaty, for example). If the later document creates a clear conflict, such as by mandating a particular activity and removing agency discretion about whether, how, and where to perform it, or by demanding such immediate action that there is simply no time to submit to the usual NEPA process, then impossibility becomes an adequate excuse for an agency's NEPA non-compliance. The instances of such "irreconcilable and fundamental" conflict are rare; agencies often assert that some partially overlapping enactment constitutes an implicit "Get out of NEPA free" card, while courts are much less permissive of that release.

In the case of variola, the only conceivable mandatory authority (other than some hypothetical new statute) would come in the form of a legally binding decision of the World Health Organization, requiring the United States to destroy the virus stockpiles by a fixed date that precluded full EIS elaboration. As indicated in chapter 5, however, the WHO, under its constituent treaty, lacks the authority to issue such binding writs upon the United States in a situation like this, so a federal agency proposing the action would still have the "discretion" to incinerate the variola samples or not—and, correspondingly, this provision does not suffice as an escape hatch from NEPA requirements.

In sum, it is unclear whether CEQ and NEPA standards would deem any proposed variola eradication measure as triggering the statutory requirements. The "impact" of the destruction would surely be minuscule in one sense: no earth would be turned, no water or air would be polluted, and the fiscal costs would be small. The physical environment would be undisturbed, other than freeing up some space in freezers and occupying a few hours of autoclave operation. However, the whole project satisfies the "controversiality" criterion— national and international debate has raged on the topic for years. Likewise, a great deal of the current dilemma centers on competing images of what the risks of retention and disposal might be and on whether, and to what extent, this decision would become a precedent for other species eradications in the future.

If some sort of NEPA full disclosure process were triggered (or if the federal government simply decided to pursue the analysis voluntarily), how much work would be entailed in satisfying the statute's procedural requirements? The first step in the undertaking is an environmental assessment (EA), a document averaging ten to fifteen pages and designed to survey the possible effects the project might have on the different categories of ecological resources. It is supposed to be multidisciplinary, engaging the relevant areas of scientific expertise, and incorporating suitable inputs from all affected governmental agencies and the public.

The EA ordinarily leads to one of two conclusions: a determination by the lead agency that there are no substantial environmental consequences worthy of further assessment (called a finding of no significant impact [FONSI]), or a determination that a full-scale environmental impact statement (EIS) is appropriate. The choice is critical: a full-blown EIS can be hundreds or thousands of pages long, requiring months or years of intensive labor, and the proposed project must be put on hold until it is completed.

In the case of variola, I suppose, there is not much that even a good faith EA or EIS could assess. The decision to destroy or preserve variola would not require exhaustive environmental research or evaluation. While the implications of the choice may be wide-ranging—as illustrated by the various chapters of this book—there is not much direct impact upon the human environment to wax poetic (or scientific) about. There are not many alternatives to consider, nor much mitigation that could be contemplated, as in the usual EIS. The potential dangers of the virus's escape from its confinement in laboratory deep freeze, the potential benefits of research upon it, and so on, could be described, but the analytical documents should be short, even if we were to include consideration of the international reverberations, specifically the corresponding destruction/preservation activities in Russia. In the same vein, while, as described in chapter 2, the variola decision may be considered precedential, in the sense that other microscopic organisms may fall under eradication consideration in the foreseeable future, in the legal sense, each of those species-specific decisions will be independent. They are thematically linked but practically autonomous, and each case will merit its own hard scrutiny, analysis, and documentation. So an EIS today would likely as a practical matter be confined to study the case of variola alone.

Still, the precedents suggest that one cannot dismiss the possibility of some type of NEPA obligations in the smallpox situation. Courts have never confronted the EA/EIS process in anything similar to this controversy, but there are suggestions in the case law about other obscure, far-flung activities that were held to require documentary analyses. For example, some form of NEPA assessment or statement was compelled in litigation regarding

the National Park Service's management program for grizzly bears in Yellowstone National Park;

the Bureau of Land Management's proposal to round up and exterminate 130 to 260 wild horses on public land in Idaho;

construction of Army facilities in Utah for testing chemical and biological warfare agents and equipment;

the Navy's proposal to capture twenty-five Atlantic bottle-nosed dolphins for deployment at a submarine base in Washington;

the National Marine Fisheries Service decision to license the capture of one hundred killer whales for permanent display or temporary scientific research; and

construction by the National Research Council of a food waste incinerator in Antarctica.

In contrast, courts have denied the necessity for full-scale NEPA operations in other close cases, such as

shipping nerve gas from Washington to Oregon;

a federal management plan to kill bison that wander outside the bounds of Yellowstone National Park;

action by the Fish and Wildlife Service to capture and bring into captivity all nine remaining wild California condors;

the Department of Agriculture's "germ plasm" preservation program for maintaining an inventory of plants and seeds;

export of nuclear-power-generating technology to the Philippines; and

movement of U.S. chemical munitions inside Germany.

This experience suggests that we could not be confident in any prediction about NEPA-related litigation regarding the smallpox virus. An individual or organizational plaintiff would, of course, have to establish adequate "standing to sue," by demonstrating a legally protected interest in the outcome, in order to invoke the jurisdiction of the federal courts. But once that hurdle has been surmounted, judges reviewing agency decisions of this sort have been instructed to give a "hard look" at the bureaucratic reasoning, holding the government to its commitment to study diverse environmental matters with care.

And that obligation includes bringing the public into the decision-making process and ensuring that environmental factors are incorporated into agency decision making at the *outset* of the process—the government has committed to studying potential environmental impacts early in its decision making, not simply inserting a boilerplate EA and FONSI into a sheaf of documents long after the "real" go-ahead for the proposal has been given. Until the environmental evaluation process is complete, the sponsoring agency is not supposed to pursue or advance the proposal in any way, including any processing of permit applications, spending money, or participating in interagency meetings designed to further the project's development. In that vein, the time to undertake an environmental study of the possible consequences of variola destruction is now, while the government is still considering the possibilities and the WHO has not yet issued a final mandate.

Beyond this fine-grained analysis of the NEPA statutory scheme, the big-picture relevance of the legislation is its overarching purpose: requiring more thoughtful, comprehensive, multidisciplinary analysis before the government makes irrevocable decisions. Even if the variola controversy gets past the formal NEPA weigh station, that philosophical mandate should still apply: the best governmental decisions (especially in situations where time is not of the essence and where we are relieved of the pressure from high-cost economic development activities) are those derived from a process that contemplates a broad range of factors, looks carefully at competing alternatives, and engages the public early on.

Another federal statute might seem more pertinent to the present challenge: the Endangered Species Act of 1973 (ESA). Like NEPA, the ESA is a landmark in environmental legislation: it is the centerpiece of biodiversity law in the United States and a compelling model for many other countries.

Also like NEPA, the ESA incorporates rhetoric and goals that are both dramatic and powerful. Congress has declared that "species of fish, wildlife, and plants are of esthetic, ecological, educational, historical, recreational, and scientific value to the Nation and its people," that "the United States has pledged itself as a sovereign state in the international community to conserve to the extent practicable the various species," and that the purpose of the enactment is to "provide a program for the conservation of such endangered species and threatened species" so "all Federal departments and agencies shall seek to conserve endangered species and threatened species and shall utilize their authorities in furtherance" of those purposes.[43]

The ambitious—some would say absolutist—goals and powers of the ESA have reflected a strong commitment to biodiversity and have earned for the statute a reputation as either a "sleeper" (for exerting an influence on public policy well beyond that foreseen by its originators) or a "giant killer" (for challenging major programs, including those attracting an impressive cadre of funders, customers, and other political partisans, and sometimes abruptly halting them in the name of preservation of an obscure endangered species and its native habitat). In the words of the U.S. Supreme Court, Congress, in this landmark legislation, determined that the value of any endangered species is "incalculable" and that "this statute was to halt and reverse the trend toward species extinction, whatever the cost."[44]

While the ESA hardly stands alone in the field of biodiversity and species conservation, it is the most powerful, the most broadly drawn, and the most likely to carry implications (or at least analogies) for variola. Its more specialized statutory cousins, focused on protecting fisheries, marine mammals, bald eagles, or other chosen creatures, are beyond the scope of this work.

But could the ESA, in principle, apply to a virus? To parse the logic of the statute's definition section requires some step-by-step examination. First, the statutory term *fish or wildlife*, which forms one of the two bases of the law's coverage, is taken to mean "any member of the animal kingdom, including without limitation any mammal, fish, bird . . . amphibian, reptile, mollusk, crustacean, arthropod, or other invertebrate."[45] Likewise, the term *plant*, the second half of the key phrase, is defined as "any member of the plant kingdom."[46] A virus fits into neither of these kingdoms, and thus appears to fall outside the statute.

Furthermore, the term *species* (which, as discussed in chapter 2, some would deem the variola to be) is not defined in a helpful manner in the act—

the explanation there is intended merely to ensure that "subspecies" and "distinct populations" would be adequately covered.[47] The definition of the term *endangered species* also contains an illuminating exception: it removes from coverage "a species of the Class Insecta determined by the Secretary to constitute a pest whose protection under the provisions of this chapter would present an overwhelming and overriding risk to man."[48] Interestingly, then, while the ESA allows groups of *insects* to be excluded from protection, there is no comparable carving out for other kinds of pests, be they microscopic or larger. The black-letter law principle of *expressio unius est exclusio alterius* (to list one item in a series is implicitly to exclude other potential items from that list) would suggest, therefore, that noninsect pests (if otherwise included in the two favored kingdoms) would be nonetheless generically protected by the statute.

Beyond that hurdle, the scope of the ESA in practice is constrained in other ways. Under the statutory scheme, the first key action is the "listing" of a species as either endangered (i.e., facing imminent extinction) or threatened (i.e., likely to become endangered in the foreseeable future). The secretary of the interior is enjoined to make determinations about listing such species "solely on the basis of the best scientific and commercial data available" and is directed to take into account "manmade factors" affecting the "continued existence" of the subject. Economic concerns (such as the cost of protecting a species) are to be excluded from consideration at this stage.

The next step in the statutory progression is the designation of a critical habitat, a geographic region to be protected from impairment or modification, in order to improve the species' chances for recovery. It is at this stage that the secretary is to take into account "the economic impact, and any other relevant impact, of specifying any particular area as critical habitat." That calculation—often requiring an ineffable cost/benefit assessment of the value of preserving a species versus the value of foregone economic development of a tract of land—has proven to be the undoing of the ESA process in many instances. Budgetary constraints have persistently impeded the secretary from protecting scores (or hundreds) of jeopardized species and habitats where competing commercial demand for the land promises new homes, highways, or jobs.

After that, the secretary is charged with developing a "recovery plan" for the species, outlining a conservation and survival program, to lead ultimately to the creature's renewal, flourishing, and delisting. A significant backlog has developed here, too, as shortages of funding and an unwillingness to face up to hard choices have meant that many listed species have languished without adequate recovery plans.

Ironically, variola would be one of the few instances in which the economic costs of ESA implementation would be minimal; that is, there would be no habitat to designate as critical. Nor would there be any particular budgetary impact on federal agencies or the private sector, no economic activities to forego if the virus were listed. No conceivable recovery plan would make sense, as variola would be confined forever to its starkly limited "environment." Other sections of the statute do prohibit anyone from possessing, selling, importing, harming, hunting, trapping, or engaging in other potentially damaging activities with respect to a listed species, but the secretary is also permitted to formulate exceptions to those constraints, for scientific purposes or to enhance the propagation or survival of the species—so the CDC employees who act to retain and experiment on the virus would be safe from prosecution.

The ESA also specifies a procedure for outsiders—who may disagree with the actions of the secretary in listing or failing to list particular species—to petition for corrective action. The law imposes a tight timetable for the government to respond to such citizen initiatives, a process for a public hearing, and the availability of judicial review of the results.

In addition, the statute provides for a senior interagency Endangered Species Committee (popularly known as the "God Squad") empowered to authorize actions that will otherwise conflict with ESA mandates, if exceptional circumstances outweigh the imperative of protecting endangered or threatened species. Two provisions related to international affairs further specify that such an exemption shall *not* be permitted if the secretary of state determines that doing so would violate a U.S. treaty obligation; and, conversely, that an appropriate warrant *shall* be granted if the secretary of defense "finds that such exemption is necessary for reasons of national security."

Finally, the regulations and case law interpreting the ESA provide a glimpse of specialized legal standards that might cast light on the variola questions. In some instances, a species may be listed and therefore protected, even though members of the imperiled race may occasionally pose a danger or threat to nearby humans and their property. For example, a protected breed of wolf may prey upon a rancher's sheep; a listed species of bear might imperil backpackers and campers near a national park. In those situations, may the aggrieved humans "take," "harm," "pursue," "shoot," or otherwise act against the predator?

The final answer to these delicate conflicts is still remarkably solicitous of the wild creatures: people are authorized to defend themselves and others from death or bodily harm (including by the use of deadly force, if necessary), but they are not permitted to hunt for even "rogue" animals. In defense of their *property*, humans are limited to means such as trying to protect a domestic herd by fencing, by repelling the aggressive creature without damaging it, or by enlisting the assistance of authorized federal agents, who may remove a hostile specimen if it poses a demonstrable threat to human safety.

The analogy to variola would be a cognate derivative of the law of self-defense. If the virus were somehow deemed within the ambit of the ESA (or if we merely decided to act as if it were), the human race would still be fully justified in its rational determination to remove the virus, and the disease of smallpox, from the human environment. We need not expose ourselves foolishly to that predation. But where it is so easy, so cheap, and so safe to preserve the species in vitro, the ethos of conservation of biodiversity should be reasserted.

Overall, the ESA, like NEPA, cannot be construed directly to regulate U.S. behavior regarding the smallpox virus. No court would find that Congress had viruses in mind when it legislated these protections for plants and animals and for the natural environment more generally. But examination of the variola case does illuminate our social commitment under ESA to species preservation, and it challenges our decisions about where to draw the line between protected and vulnerable life forms. Why do we extend special recognition to big creatures and not to small? Why are we more solicitous about dramatic, evocative entities than about the commonplace or invisible? Why do we draw such arbitrary lines between "living" things and others?

If the ESA preaches that all life is sacred, what are its parameters—in social impact, even if not in precise legislative coverage? Pondering these questions, even if there is a mismatch between existing statutes and the variola problem at hand, can provide a philosophical base that should assist refinement of public policy in each sphere.

CONCLUSION

In sum, the law of environmental protection—both its international and its domestic U.S. applications—is not directly relevant to the question of extermination of the variola virus. This body of law and policy is still too young and underdeveloped to address issues of such novelty and peculiarity.

At the same time, however, the ethos and animating spirit behind that emerging corpus of law—the assertion of a deep compatibility between humans and nature; the insistence on implementing a strategy for planning human activities in a sustainable, respectful fashion; and especially the appreciation for the value of, and the threats to, biodiversity—are instructive. As the Supreme Court has noted, genetic variations should be husbanded as potential resources: "They are the keys to puzzles which we cannot solve, and may provide answers to questions which we have not yet learned to ask."[49] The call from other commentators to "judge every scrap of biodiversity as priceless while we learn to use it and come to understand what it means to humanity" strikes a deep chord, even if it was drafted with creatures other than a virus in mind.[50] The environmental dimension of the smallpox story, therefore, calls upon us to consider the fate of variola with a sensitivity to its posture within the grand scheme of nature and a humility about humanity's approach to it.

CHAPTER 5

THE WORLD HEALTH ORGANIZATION

This chapter investigates the contributions that international and domestic organizations have made to the smallpox story. It therefore combines aspects of institutional history, political culture, law, and organizational behavior, to recount the world's complex involvement with variola from yet another perspective. Most attention is paid here to the World Health Organization, the moving force in the decades-long drama, but aspects of internal U.S. government decision making are also discussed for additional insight.[1]

The World Health Organization (WHO) is the parent institution for global cooperation in pursuit of "a state of complete physical, mental, and social well-being, and not merely the absence of disease and infirmity."[2] It has long played the starring role in the human efforts surrounding smallpox, from disease control to eradication. It is the WHO that has repeatedly directed, and then repeatedly delayed, the disposal of the final variola stockpiles.

The World Health Organization is a creature of law, created by treaty and governed by its constitution and other internal rules. Understanding its powers and limitations, and its role in international health affairs, is fundamental to a complete portrait of the variola eradication decisions, so this chapter presents an overview of the organization, its legal personality and capacity, and what it has said and done regarding the virus inventories.

THE W.H.O.: DESCRIPTION AND POWERS

The WHO is one of the sixteen "specialized agencies" of the United Nations. It was created by treaty as an independent entity after World War II, but its roots and its efforts to fulfill the global health mandate go back much further.

The earliest precursors of modern international health organizations were, on a regional level, the International Sanitary Bureau established in 1902 (and which later evolved into the Pan American Sanitary Bureau and ultimately into the Pan American Health Organization); and, on a global level, the Office International d'Hygiène Publique (OIHP), created in 1907 by twelve countries and headquartered in Paris. The OIHP grew to encompass nearly sixty countries at the outbreak of World War I, and after the war it developed an indirect relationship with the League of Nations Health Organization. The OIHP served to supervise the improvement of quarantine procedures, to publicize outbreaks of dangerous diseases, and to collect reports on emerging epidemics. Smallpox was one of a handful of communicable illnesses of special concern to the organization.

After World War II, the new United Nations Economic and Social Council (one of six organs of the UN system) called for the creation of a new global health organization. A treaty to create the WHO was quickly drawn up and signed, and it entered into force on April 7, 1948, when it was ratified by the necessary twenty-six UN member states. That anniversary is now marked annually as World Health Day. The WHO—the first specialized agency so created—concluded a formal relationship agreement with the United Nations in July 1948.

The United States, which had not joined the interwar League of Nations or its specialized health arm, did not hesitate long in affiliating with the new World Health Organization, ratifying the constitution on June 21, 1948. In the process, the U.S. Senate insisted upon attaching two legally binding "reservations," thereby retaining for the United States the right to withdraw from the organization (an issue upon which the organic charter was silent) and declaring that nothing in the WHO constitution required the United States to enact any specific legislative program. While these provisos might have posed an important challenge to the inclusiveness of the WHO and to its legislative powers, the organization's credentials committee was, according to Javed Siddiqi, "undisturbed" by the American assertions, and they have not proven of much operational importance in the practical life of the institution.

Today, membership in the WHO has swollen to 191, embracing virtually every country in all inhabited portions of the planet, irrespective of national ideology, degree of economic development, or range of health challenges to be faced. The organization's structure is decentralized; member states are organized into six somewhat unconventional, highly autonomous regions, with area offices covering Africa, the Americas, Southeast Asia, Europe, the Eastern Mediterranean, and the Western Pacific. Like many other modern international organizations, the WHO maintains an internal governance structure featuring three key organs: the assembly, the executive board, and the secretariat.

The World Health Assembly (WHA) is the basic legislative body of the WHO. All member countries are represented. The assembly meets annually in May, usually at the WHO headquarters in Geneva. Its main functions are to approve the biennial program of operations (and the associated budget) and to resolve major policy issues. Its formal pronouncements, the World Health Assembly Resolutions, have been the major vehicle for global expression and determinations on smallpox, as examined below.

The executive board comprises thirty-two individuals, typically technical experts in a variety of health-related specialties, designated by specified member states who are elected by the WHA for three-year terms. The executive board meets twice a year (January and May) and functions as the executive organ, carrying out the determinations of the assembly and providing leadership to help shape future WHO actions.

The secretariat, headed by a director-general (currently Dr. Gro Harlem Brundtland, former prime minister of Norway), is composed of 3,800 health and other experts, housed at the Geneva headquarters, in the six regional offices, and in the field. The staff of international civil servants is obligated to serve the organization, not their home governments; they are not "representatives" of their respective countries of origin.

The functions and objectives of the WHO are as varied as the stresses upon global health and well-being. Under its organic constitution, the objective of the WHO is nothing less than "the attainment by all peoples of the highest possible level of health." As needs demand and circumstances permit, the organization exercises the responsibility to, among other things:

assist national governments in strengthening their internal health systems;

maintain highest quality technical services in areas such as epidemiology;

promote cooperation among scientific and professional groups to contribute to the enhancement of health;

develop international standards for food, biological, and pharmaceutical products;

provide emergency aid during times of crisis;

establish a standardized international nomenclature of diseases;

and, of special interest to the current inquiry,

stimulate work to prevent and control epidemic, endemic, and other diseases and

promote and coordinate biomedical and health services research.

To enable that grandiose agenda, the WHO draws upon two primary sources of funds. First, the regular budget consists of assessed contributions from member states, roughly following the general United Nations scale of dues. For the two-year period 2000 to 2001, this account totaled $842.654 million. (In fact, this portion of the WHO budget has been frozen at that level for several years, in response to many countries, especially the United States, pushing for zero real growth in the budgets of international organizations.) In addition, the organization receives substantial voluntary contributions from states and other sources, known as extra budgetary contributions, which were budgeted at $1.097 billion for that biennium. The total funds available to the organization, therefore, were $1,939,654,000.[3]

In any account of the WHO's major successes, pride of place is always given to the eradication of smallpox. This was surely the organization's finest hour, and it provides the template that its partisans hope to apply to other diseases, from polio to measles to guinea worm disease. Sexually transmitted diseases, HIV/AIDS in particular, have become a major focus of WHO activities, as have tuberculosis, leprosy, malaria, and the newly emerging hemorrhagic fevers such as Ebola. Other WHO activities under the rubric of "Health for all by the year 2000" have included increased access to vaccinations, opposition to tobacco use, and an "Expanded Programme on Immunizations" for the leading childhood diseases. The WHO also maintains a "strike force" of trained experts who can be dispatched within twenty-four hours to the site of a new disease outbreak, to provide skilled assistance to the victims and to the local first responders.

More broadly, the WHO has taken on the mandate to try to improve global well-being in basic ways, by promoting healthy lifestyles and environments, ensuring access to safe drinking water and nutrition, and informing the public about mechanisms for avoiding inherent health risks. The WHO is also responsible for setting international standards to ensure the highest quality of biological and pharmaceutical preparations and for ensuring that laboratories dealing with infectious materials work under safe conditions.

The WHO also collaborates closely with other institutions within the UN family, including UNICEF (e.g., on promoting "baby friendly hospitals"), the World Bank (e.g., on funding AIDS research), and the International Labor Organization (e.g., on programs to promote chemical safety in the workplace). In addition, the WHO maintains official relations with 180 nongovernmental organizations (NGOs) and leverages their contributions to supplement a variety of programs (e.g., Rotary International's support for the global polio eradication campaign). Moreover, nearly 1,200 leading health-related institutions around the world have been designated as WHO Collaborating Centers, cooperating in a wide range of health research, testing, and other operations.[4] The WHO is further assisted by expert advisory panels—in a recent year there were at least fifty-four such committees, encompassing some 2,000 experts in many specialties.[5]

Of course, the WHO is not without its critics. There have been, from time to time, serious allegations that the organization is bureaucratically top-heavy, poorly organized, unfocused on its core missions, overly optimistic in its health projections, profligate, and politicized in the same way that other United Nations entities have sometimes been.[6] As Allyn Lise Taylor has argued, a "conservative organizational culture" inhibits the institution's ability to assume a more assertive posture on even the most pressing health issues or to demand greater funding and support.[7] Observers have charged that the WHO has not been successful in forging a genuine global alliance for mobilizing the funding commitments necessary to make the organization's adoption of "Health for all" into a genuine strategy and not merely empty rhetoric.

The World Health Organization, cognizant of the sovereign perquisites of its member states, serves the international health community in a variety of ways, defined by its institutional powers and capabilities. As a first lawmaking power, the World Health Assembly has quasilegislative authority to adopt, via a two-thirds vote, regulations on important technical matters specified in the WHO constitution. Once adopted, such a regulation is legally binding upon all member countries (even those that disavowed it in the assembly and voted against it), except those that specifically notify the WHO that they reject the regulation or accept it only with certain reservations. Even then, an objecting state's reservation must be accepted by the assembly before it can become effective.

These International Health Regulations (IHR) empower the WHO to introduce uniform technical specifications regarding quarantine requirements; nomenclature for diseases and public health practices; criteria for diagnostic procedures; safety, purity, and potency of biological and pharmaceutical products; and advertising and labeling of biological and pharmaceutical materials. More than two hundred such standards now exist, and more than one hundred collaborating laboratories assist in implementing them.

The concept of enabling the WHO to act in this direct, legally binding manner was based on the assessment that creating new mandatory standards through the ordinary mechanism of international law—that is, through a sequence of treaties, each of which would have to be signed and ratified (usually with the concomitant delays of legislative approval) by each member state—was too slow, piecemeal, and uncertain to serve in the fast-breaking world of infectious diseases. The streamlined process transfers some considerable authority to the WHO, while still allowing a recalcitrant country to "contract out" of a provision it cannot abide.

The leading application of IHR concerns monitoring outbreaks of diseases of international concern. One of the WHO's primary functions is surveillance: it serves as the world's health "alarm bell," notifying the community about dangerous eruptions of communicable diseases. As increased mobility of people, expansion of international trade in foodstuffs and other biological materials, and the growing adaptability of pathogens have all contributed to an ever-more-complex global health portrait, the WHO serves as the "network of net-works," linking local, regional, national, and international health-reporting systems, via both formal and informal communications. The organization also provides the most authoritative standards of reference for defining diseases and classifying specimens and for ensuring that member states maintain adequate health resources, programs, and organizations to fulfill their obligations to enforce the international surveillance, quarantine, and other standards.

Under the IHR, states have three types of obligations: (1) to notify the world community when an outbreak occurs in one of the diseases of special international significance; (2) to maintain prescribed sanitary conditions, health services, and trained personnel at national borders (especially airports and sea-ports); and (3) to develop health measures and procedures regulating international travel and transportation that are no more burdensome than necessary in constraining the conveyance of possibly infectious persons and goods.

However, the current IHR on disease reporting are a starkly limited tool. As David P. Fidler has pointed out, the organization has largely allowed the regulations to deteriorate as a framework for control of the most worrisome infectious diseases.[8] First, the IHR are confined, at present, to only three diseases: plague, cholera, and yellow fever. (Smallpox used to be covered but was dropped when incidence of the disease was eliminated globally.) Worse, they are incompletely complied with: many countries, fearing negative impacts on their tourism or exports, fail to provide accurate, comprehensive, timely data. Conversely, other states have frequently erected health-related barriers to trade that inhibit commerce and travel more tightly than necessary. In addition, the mechanics of the reporting system are antiquated, not yet adapted to modern social institutions and communications methods.

In 1995 the WHO began to upgrade the IHR. Provisional and amended drafts of a thorough revision have been distributed and extensive comments taken into account; progress, not surprisingly, is slow. An experimental pilot project in twenty-one countries features prompt electronic reporting of many different diseases and clinical syndromes of interest, providing data to alert local and other health officials.

In addition to having that type of legislative or rule-making authority, the assembly has a broad power to negotiate and adopt international treaties on behalf of the WHO. While such an agreement would not be automatically bind-ing upon any member that declines to ratify it, each member must take deci-sive action within eighteen months, leading to acceptance by its government. If the home government fails to adopt or ratify the agreement, it must report to the WHO the reasons for nonacceptance. To date, no such treaties have been concluded; the first, a multilateral framework convention concerning tobacco production and sales, is still under development, and is proving controversial.

The most frequently exercised power of the World Health Organization is its issuance of non–legally binding recommendations to member states "with respect to any matter within the competence of the Organization." Each mem-ber is obligated to "report annually on the action taken with respect to recom-mendations made to it." This has become the most effective tool of the assem-bly: to exert its scientific leadership and its moral suasion to guide member countries to accept its direction.

Influenza surveillance is a leading illustration of the success of the WHO system. Some 110 national and independent laboratories in eighty-three coun-tries continuously monitor local flu outbreaks, providing rapid, authoritative assessment of infectious patterns and the emergence of new viral strains. Information from those disparate sources is fed into four WHO Collaborating Centers for Influenza, which develop recommendations for the three viral strains to be included in the next season's influenza vaccine, a lifesaving pre-caution for many.

In sum, then, the World Health Organization, as a modern, assertive, and essential international organization, possesses a combination of both legal and political powers. In some areas, covered by the International Health Regula-tions, it has been delegated the authority to make law, binding upon its mem-bership. These concern a range of public health issues, enabling international cooperation in complex and urgent antidisease efforts. Even there, however, countries mostly retain the sovereign right to dodge obligations.

The members of the WHO are independent countries who have, for the most part, demonstrated little affinity for transferring a substantial amount of national sovereignty to international institutions. This is not like the European Union, where sovereign states have consciously ceded incremental bits of their autonomy irrevocably to continentwide supragovernmental authorities. Maybe that kind of unity will come someday in the field of global public health—the enhancement of the IHR and a streamlined rule-making process would seem to be tentative steps in that direction. But at the moment, the genuine legal capabilities of the organization are limited, at best.

The political muscle of the organization, however, is more comprehensive. The scientific resources that the WHO can bring to bear, as well as its impressive institutional memory and the ability to mount technical and financial assistance programs, ensure its clout in an increasingly interdependent world. The WHO's history of struggling to reach broad international consensus—sometimes revisiting certain issues for years in order to achieve scientific and political harmony—helps bolster the weight of its pronouncements (if not always their timeliness). The WHO has earned the right to be taken seriously, including by the most powerful countries, and its authoritative voice on public health matters routinely moves even the most hard-nosed political leaders.

The WHO must, however, be careful not to overplay its hand. The organization has no power to enforce compliance, to mandate any particular resolution of a dispute, or to impose sanctions upon recalcitrant states. As noted below, virtually all the assembly's and the executive board's actions regarding smallpox eradication and variola destruction have been phrased as recommendations or requests, not as orders. The Geneva officials operate through the tools of persuasion, and when they earnestly urge countries to do something, the countries do pay heed but are not legally compelled to obey.

WHAT HAS THE W.H.O. DONE ABOUT SMALLPOX?

The World Health Organization's record regarding smallpox is long and distinguished but also characterized by erratic zigzags at crucial moments when the eradication question has ripened. Starting in the early and mid-1950s, as early as its third annual meeting, the World Health Assembly, prompted by the executive board, had attempted to standardize smallpox vaccines, had commissioned the study of a global campaign against smallpox, had urged national authorities to make smallpox eradication a priority, and had articulated the modification of international travelers' certificates of smallpox vaccination.

By 1958, the assembly had launched a "programme having as its objective the eradication of smallpox," and in 1967, as discussed in chapter 1, it "intensified" that global campaign. By 1976, as success in that monumental enterprise came within sight, the assembly began to turn its attention to the aftermath, specifically the question of variola stockpiles. It requested "all governments and laboratories to cooperate fully in preparing an international registry of laboratories retaining stocks of variola virus but, at the same time, urges all laboratories which do not require such stocks of variola virus to destroy them." The next step, in 1977, was to request that variola specimens should continue to be held only by WHO collaborating centers, under conditions of maximum safety.

In May 1980, the WHO was finally able to declare "solemnly that the world and all its peoples have won freedom from smallpox." The assembly then endorsed the recommendations of the Global Commission for the Certification of Smallpox Eradication, including the discontinuation of smallpox vaccination of ordinary civilians and the suspension of the requirement for international certification of vaccination for international travelers. Other recommendations included number 9: "No more than four WHO collaborating centres should be approved as suitable to hold, and handle, stocks of variola virus" and number 10: "Other laboratories should be asked to destroy any stocks of variola virus that they hold, or transfer them to an approved WHO collaborating centre."[9]

In the succeeding years, events progressed largely as anticipated. Routine smallpox vaccination of civilians was terminated by all countries; substantial reserve stocks of smallpox vaccine were maintained by the WHO and by several individual states; the known variola stocks were concentrated in only two facilities (the Centers for Disease Control in Atlanta, and the Research Institute for Viral Preparations in Moscow); and advances in genetic research parsed many of the secrets of different strains of variola DNA.

Attention then turned increasingly to the question of disposal or maintenance of the reserved variola stocks. In 1985, the WHO Committee on Orthopoxvirus Infections surveyed sixty virologists in academia and public health in twenty-one countries; only five held the view that variola should be retained indefinitely; any necessary research, most of the experts felt, could continue adequately on the basis of nonexpressing (i.e., noninfectious) cloned residues. In October 1986, the committee itself unanimously recommended that the stocks should be destroyed.

In December 1990, a subsequent group, the Ad Hoc Committee on Orthopoxvirus Infections, confirmed the eradication recommendation, and proposed a deadline of December 31, 1993, for carrying out the destruction. However, a significant debate on the issue had emerged within the scientific community and the general public, and the question was revisited at the Ninth International Congress of Virology in Glasgow, Scotland, in August 1993. The ad hoc committee met a second time in September 1994 and aired arguments for and against eradication (see chapters 7 and 8 for an expanded discussion of those considerations), as well as assessed the opinions of expert and professional groups. The ad hoc committee was again unanimous that all variola stocks should be destroyed in the autoclaves, but there was disagreement as to precisely when this final elimination should occur. Eight of the ten members favored June 30, 1995; the remaining two would have postponed the action for five years.[10]

In fact, all those dates passed without dispositive action by the WHO bodies. In January 1995, the executive board postponed consideration of the ad hoc committee's report, but in January 1996, the executive board voted to recommend destruction on June 30, 1999, with the additional delay to be used to achieve a broader consensus for the irreversible action. At its May 25, 1996, meeting, the assembly concurred with that judgment, subject to confirmation by yet another assembly vote prior to the expiration of the moratorium.

At that point, the action reverted to the ad hoc committee, which met for its third session in January 1999 to review once again the merits of the proposal, in light of recent technical and epidemiological events. This time, the ad hoc committee was deeply divided: five members favored proceeding with destruction by the June 1999 deadline; two favored eventual destruction, but subject to another five-year moratorium; and two others favored indefinite retention.[11] At the same time, a survey of WHO member states revealed that seventy-four supported destruction of the virus under the established timetable, four were undecided, and one was against destruction—a result that at first appeared to display a broad global consensus, until the numbers were unpacked, revealing that the four "undecided" members were Britain, France, Italy, and the United States, and the sole dissenter was Russia.

With some drama, on May 24, 1999, the World Health Assembly again "punted" the issue into the future. While strongly reaffirming the decision to destroy the variola virus eventually, the assembly noted a lack of consensus as to when that action should occur and decided "to authorize temporary retention up to not later than 2002," subject to annual review, for the purposes of allowing further international research into antiviral agents and improved vaccines and of permitting high-priority investigation into the genetic structure and pathogenesis of variola. In the assembly, twenty-seven countries cosponsored the compromise resolution calling for the deferral, and twenty-five countries spoke in favor, with no dissenting views. Some member states, notably Japan and India, but also Iran, Nicaragua, and Zambia, were unhappy with the delay, succumbing only to substantial behind-the-scenes lobbying and diplomatic pressure.

In December 1999, the WHO convened a sixteen-member Advisory Committee on Variola Virus Research, charged with developing and overseeing a research plan for priority work on the virus, preparatory to implementation of the final eradication. This body outlined an ambitious set of objectives for the scientific inquiries but resolutely asserted that the moratorium from final destruction of the stocks "should, under no circumstances, continue beyond the end of 2002."[12]

Events soon proved the undoing of that "final" commitment. By the end of 2001, it was clear that the aggressive program of research could not be completed by the projected date; the constellation of political forces was also radically altered by the September 11 terrorism and by the Bush administration's decision not to proceed with the variola destruction program as scheduled. The advisory committee reluctantly reversed course and concluded that the December 2002 deadline should be extended yet again, to allow "essential research" to proceed. The WHO director-general concurred in that judgment, suggesting that the scientific inquiries should continue apace and that the assembly might revisit the variola destruction question in two or three years. In January 2002, the executive board, too, bowed to the inevitable, and recommended that the assembly, at its May 2002 session, concede to another deferral of the long-awaited autoclaving. Some countries resisted the migration toward a new lease on life for variola, but the assembly eventually acquiesced, permitting a "time-limited and periodically reviewed" research program and anticipating that "a proposed new date for destruction should be set when the research accomplishments and outcomes allow consensus to be reached."[13]

WHAT ARE THE CURRENT VARIOLA STOCKS?

The biological material at the center of the variola controversy is, in one sense, remarkably unimposing and ill-defined. As late as 1999, the virus samples held by the CDC in Atlanta, for example, were not well categorized; little clinical data about the individual strains had been collected and retained. No pathogenicity studies had been conducted on the specimens, and their viability had not been systematically checked. Live virus had been successfully grown from three of the samples, but some contamination was also observed. No physical examination of the repository had been undertaken to confirm the complete inventory.

The 120 samples held by the Vector laboratory in Koltsovo were also poorly understood. Work had been done on relative pathogenicity, and different strains clearly carried different properties, but clinical data associated with each specimen were limited. Moreover, no one knew how much overlap there might be between the two national laboratories' respective holdings. The WHO did not have an active inventory of other laboratories around the world that might hold cloned DNA fragments of the virus (at least five of these facilities were known), nor were transfers of such materials routinely reported.

Similarly, uncertainty pervaded the estimates of the world's holdings of smallpox vaccine and of vaccinia immune globulin (VIG) (for treating adverse reactions to the vaccine). There were formal registries of up to sixty to ninety million doses of vaccine, but the status, storage conditions, and continuing viability of much of that inventory was unknown (and often doubtful).[14]

One piece of early good news came from the WHO director-general: inspection teams dispatched in October 1999 and February 2000 assayed the biological safety and physical security of the collaborating centers in Atlanta and Novosibirsk. They found, to the relief (and surprise) of many, that the variola inventories were protected by "fully satisfactory" mechanisms and procedures, allaying fears that dated back to the inadequate conditions prevalent when the Russian stocks were held at the antiquated Moscow facility.

World Health Organization members, anticipating a possible legal controversy if the concerned countries are unable to speak with one voice on the final disposition of the samples, had also inquired about legal "ownership" of the stocks. The virulent materials had been originally collected and dispatched to the two collaborating centers from a variety of countries, public and private laboratories, and individuals. The documents that accompanied the transfers were typically short and ambiguous on questions of the parties' reserved rights, and some of the paperwork has not been retained. Commentators since that time have been contradictory and confused about various stakeholders' legal rights. What would happen if a sending country and its collaborating center were to differ about the fate of a sample—whose legal rights would prevail? The WHO legal staff was able to conclude only that the materials had been left with the collaborating centers for safekeeping under the supervision of the WHO, and "ownership therefore remained unclear."[15]

SMALLPOX RESEARCH

The 1999 advisory committee was precise in determining which variola-related research activities should be permitted; it reviewed the findings and conclusions of numerous predecessor investigators, including prior WHO committees and national bodies such as the 1999 report of the U.S. Institute of Medicine.

The first priority was collecting precise DNA sequence information on additional variola strains, beyond those already more or less comprehensively mapped. An associated task would be comparisons of isolates from different regions, years, or persons. As technology advances, and as the genome-sequencing chore becomes quicker and easier, additional scientific value might be extracted, providing insights of relevance not only to poxviruses, but far more generally.

The major public health aspects of the research agenda focused, as had previous inquiries, on vaccines, chemotherapeutic agents, and chemoprophylactic agents. The search for a safer, but equally efficacious, smallpox vaccine was stressed, and several different strategies for vaccine development were to be assessed, although the difficulty of securing approval from national regulatory authorities to test and market any such treatment would be daunting. The committee reported that investigation of four candidate therapeutic drugs had been discouraging to date, but there was somewhat greater promise for two potential prophylactic treatments. Some on the committee asserted that improved vaccines were likely to be more attainable, and would substantially mitigate the necessity for postexposure treatments. Among the proffered antiviral drugs were some (such as cidofovir) that were already routinely used for combating other viruses and seemed to have some effectiveness in vitro against variola—but research so far had been limited only to exploitation of existing drugs, rather than discovery of new compounds.

As with prior expert committees, this group also concluded that improved diagnostic and detection capabilities should be pursued, even though developing these novel capabilities would require sustained access to live, intact variola virus. The possibility that variola could serve as a model for basic research into human immunity and infection was also intriguing, although the committee would not warrant open-ended, fundamental research as a justification for preserving variola indefinitely.

In its first three progress reports, through December 2001, the WHO Advisory Committee noted achievements in several areas. First, regarding assessment of the existing stockpile, the committee reported that the CDC holds 451 viral isolates; of these, 49 (based on geographical source, year of isolation, etc.) were selected for analysis and 45 of those proved viable. Russian samples were not yet as thoroughly evaluated, but many have likewise been found to be viable, including 23 strains selected from among 50 that were not present in the American collection. The two laboratories had begun to cooperate and coordinate their activities (which could also help ameliorate a persistent shortage of funding at Vector).[16]

The WHO committee also noted approvingly that the research plan was moving forward simultaneously toward several accomplishments: A number of different technologies had been described for real-time detection and identification of variola virus and prompt diagnosis of smallpox infection. The nucleotide sequences of at least ten variola virus strains (nine of *Variola major*, one of *Variola minor*) were now substantially known, a success achieved more rapidly than originally contemplated, and additional gene sequencing (concentrating on samples from more diverse kinds of materials) was under way. Research on new vaccines, drawing on alternatives to the intact vaccinia virus, was encouraging, but far from complete.[17]

The leading candidate antiviral medication, cidofovir, had continued to fare well in in vitro tests, and would progress soon to consideration in animal models. It is also being pursued for the status of an investigational new drug with the U.S. Food and Drug Administration on an expedited timetable to facilitate its experimentation and possible use in a smallpox emergency. At the same time, this drug, too, has its limitations—it can cause kidney damage, it must be administered via injection, instead of as an aerosol, and it costs $700 per dose. In addition, some 270 other antiviral compounds have been screened in cell cultures for activity against variola, and 140 have been selected for additional evaluation. In support of those inquiries, researchers have made considerable progress in developing a suitable animal model (a smallpoxlike disease in cynomolgus monkeys) for evaluating countervariola drugs.[18]

Noteworthy institutional achievements are also taking place, if not always as quickly as we might hope. A dedicated Poxvirus Bioinformatics Resource Center and a National Electronic Disease Surveillance System have been established, and the CDC is creating a specialized sequencing and bioinformatics laboratory for this effort. Overall, however, the committee concluded—and the director-general corroborated—that additional research, including investigations requiring access to intact, viable variola virus, will need to continue beyond 2002 in order to accomplish the ambitious objectives established by the assembly and its members.

THE EFFECTS OF SEPTEMBER 11

In the wake of the September 11, 2001, terrorist attacks, the entire range of counterterrorist research activities assumed new urgency, and antivariola inquiries have been no exception. Increasingly, experts concurred that smallpox was "the single most dangerous raw material for a non-nuclear terror attack" and second only to anthrax as a prominent worry for civil defense authorities.[19] The World Health Organization, like the United States and others, focused greater energies on variola, and reviewed models of hypothetical smallpox releases in order to determine more accurately how much vaccine would be necessary to contain an outbreak. The WHO also updated and released a new iteration of its flagship publication, Health Aspects of Biological and Chemical Weapons, in the effort to arm the global community with frank but nonhysterical assessments of the emerging threats.

In November 2001, the U.S. government abruptly reversed its course on variola eradication, in a manner that directly and unilaterally conflicted with the WHO's guidance. Responding to the attacks in September and the anthrax bioterrorism in October, the Bush administration announced that it would not proceed with the destruction of the variola inventory until researchers had accomplished a series of demanding objectives. These ambitious goals far surpassed the scope approved by the WHO and would take far longer than December 2002 to accomplish—some say that at least a decade of additional investigation and development would be required.

The new American position was that variola should be retained until the successful development of (1) a new vaccine, free of the adverse side effects of vaccinia and therefore safe for the entire community; (2) two antiviral pharmaceuticals, which attack variola via independent biological pathways; (3) "sniffers" capable of timely detection of variola in the environment; (4) improved diagnostic procedures for identifying smallpox infection in the human body; and (5) a capability for counteracting genetically engineered variants of the variola virus.

Lev Sandakhchiev, the director of the Vector laboratory where Russia's variola samples are held, immediately welcomed the decision as promoting research necessary for the United States, Russia, and the whole world. As noted, the WHO director-general in December 2001, and the executive board in January 2002, concurred in the removal of the December 2002 deadline. The next move—conceding an open-ended permission for research, without the establishment of another "final" target date—was reluctantly accepted by the World Health Assembly in May 2002.

WHY IS THIS TAKING SO LONG?

Even by the standards of international organizations, which tend to proceed at a stately pace, the World Health Organization's dialogues about smallpox have been greatly extended. More than twenty years have passed since the last case of the disease anywhere on earth; the level of scientific research on the viral samples has long been (at least until recently) quite moderate. The world, overwhelmed by new, more puzzling viral threats such as the Ebola, Marburg, and West Nile viruses, has largely turned its attention elsewhere.

Fifteen years have now elapsed since the first WHO committee resolutely, and unanimously, called for variola's eradication, and the first proposed deadline—December 31, 1993—has receded into history. The other self-imposed target dates—June 30, 1995, and June 30, 1999, and most recently December 31, 2002—turned into nonevents, as the search for an elusive global consensus has proceeded. For a world community that so emphatically and repeatedly declares its commitment to destruction of variola, as a crescendo for the triumphant human struggle against smallpox, it seems to be taking an inordinately long time to flip the switch on the autoclaves.

Surely the complexity of the underlying justifications and rebuttals in the variola destruction debate, presented in chapters 7 and 8, provides the main reason for the WHO's difficulty in speaking with one consistent voice on this question. But politics, too, has always played a role in smallpox matters, and it is instructive to explore here domestic and international issues as opaque as bureaucratic turf, budgets, raw power, and honest differences in perspective on the critical variables.

THE U.S. AND OTHER PERSPECTIVES

The United States, it must be noted at the outset, has vacillated as much as any other country or international organization on this question. In May 1990, for example, the secretary of Health and Human Services (HHS), Louis Sullivan, declared that "there is no scientific reason not to destroy the remaining stock of the wild virus." He promised to eliminate the U.S. variola inventory (after DNA sequencing of the genome had been completed) and led the U.S. effort in support of prompt global eradication.[20] That posture was sustained for a few years, but later in the decade, his successor at HHS, Donna Shalala, was in the forefront in lobbying other WHO delegations to delay that final step in order to permit additional scientific research on measures to counter the growing threat of terrorist use of a biological weapon.[21] At the same time, the private U.S. citizens who sit in their personal capacities on the WHO's ad hoc committee voted unanimously to support prompt destruction.[22]

Behind the scenes lies a story of incessant interagency wrangling on the issue, with HHS (in support of destruction) engaged in a winner-take-all battle with the Department of Defense (seeking to preserve the virus, for reasons elaborated in succeeding chapters). This split was managed, or perhaps exacerbated, by the National Security Council staff, which sometimes played the "honest broker" role in mediating between the competing perspectives, while sometimes putting a forceful thumb on the scales on the side of destruction. Meanwhile, both the Department of State (potentially a key player in any controversy touching upon international relations) and the U.S. Arms Control and Disarmament Agency (for most of this period, the lead federal agency for the weapons-control negotiations and policy aspects of the smallpox question) remained quiescent, or at least did not play major roles.[23] Congress, too, got involved, for example, in the form of a March 22, 1999, letter to President Bill Clinton from seven Republican senators, urging retention of the variola stockpile to permit biodefense research.

The ultimate position of the U.S. government in 1995, a convoluted resolution of the competing political interests, at least temporarily or halfheartedly supported the HHS logic. But the 1999 phase of the struggle saw a reversal, widely interpreted as a victory (albeit perhaps just as short-lived) for the Pentagon. The 2001 about-face was reportedly the result of an unanimous interagency committee studying bioterrorism issues more generally, but it, too, was expected to generate the usual quantity of internal and external dissension.

Other countries, too, have been internally conflicted about this dilemma, usually replicating the American alignment of interests: the ministry of defense arguing for retention and the civilian counterparts pressing for prompt eradication. Great Britain has played a particularly active role, being almost single-handedly responsible for initiating the delay in definitive WHO action in 1995. Australia, Japan, India, and Mexico, among others, have from time to time exerted leadership in one direction or the other. A variety of economically developing countries—including many who had suffered most recently from the disease—were vigorous proponents of prompt incineration of the last smallpox residues.

Some of these skeptics worry that all the attention and resources devoted to smallpox could divert the world's attention from their health agendas. For example, will the WHO and its members be as diligent in exploring a solution to the AIDS crisis, if scarce funding is diverted into variola inquiries? If efficacious vaccines and antivirals are developed, will they be allocated to needy consumers strictly on a market basis, or will the poor countries manage to avoid being shut out of the high-stakes and high-cost pharmaceuticals?

As noted above, at the turn of the century, the overwhelming majority of WHO member countries had consistently expressed their support for variola destruction but were cajoled into waiting. And some voices occasionally support the notion that if the variola stocks are to be preserved, even temporarily, they should be housed in some sort of international facility, perhaps located in a neutral country and directly supervised by the WHO, instead of remaining within the United States and Russia.[24] No one knows what such a multilateral institution would look like, and there are few promising models. Who would control the activities; how would the benefits be distributed; and how would it balance competing imperatives for openness (so all could be confident that the laboratory would be free from weapons-related work) and for security (so no one could pilfer research accomplishments and bend them to unilateral military or commercial advantage)?

One outcome of the ongoing WHO-supervised shared research enterprise has been to further cement the nascent pattern of cooperation between the two former cold war rivals. In agreeing to seek postponement of any WHO resolution on the eradication question, the United States and Russia found themselves pursuing avenues for additional scientific collaboration and joint biological research at a time when their bilateral relationship was otherwise increasingly strained. White House officials, while maintaining that the American position had been developed purely on the basis of national security and scientific considerations, were quick to note that it also opened additional opportunities for international cooperation. The United States has stepped up its investment in joint bioterrorism-related research with Russia, particularly with the Vector laboratory, and that collaboration is already beginning to pay off. Cooperative smallpox-related research, therefore, might provide a useful vehicle for the two military giants to harmonize their efforts and together demonstrate a measure of leadership for the rest of the world.

CONCLUSION

The World Health Organization cannot compel the United States and Russia to conform to its decisions, restrictions, and timetables for variola research and elimination. The scope of the WHO's legal authorities is restricted; its mandatory powers in this area do not extend beyond the ability to issue recommendations, requests, and guidance. In their determinations about smallpox, the assembly and executive board have been careful to lead by persuasion and influence, not exceeding their legal prowess. America's newfound resistance to variola destruction can doubtless succeed, if the United States (and Russia) stay firmly on the new course. The WHO, like other modern international organizations, is not a true "democracy." Although the principle of "one country, one vote" is firmly enshrined in the operating rules of the assembly and the executive board, the political culture of the institution tells a different story. While the United States and Russia cannot always dictate the WHO's course of action, the fact that they are the most powerful protagonists—and especially that they continue as physical custodians of the only known, WHO-sanctioned stocks of variola virus—grant them the leading roles.

On the other hand, even the military giants would be reluctant to ignore the world's leading health institution and its expertise. The political, technical, and moral weight of the WHO—earned through years of exemplary service in combating the disease, researching its causative agent, and safeguarding the world against its resurgence—compels deference. On the question of variola eradication, world public opinion has been approaching unanimity; the two possessory countries would doubtless incur a significant political cost to resist it indefinitely.

At this point, the institutional dimension of the smallpox story suggests that the United States and Russia face something of a "use it or lose it" mandate. That is, the rationales for continued possession—that additional research is needed on improved vaccines, novel antivirals, and sophisticated detectors— wear thin for many international observers, who have heard the same song for some years, largely unaccompanied by dedication of serious funding or effort. Only recently—when confronted by the "final" extension of the eradication date to December 31, 2002—have the Centers for Disease Control and the Vector laboratory truly undertaken an energetic research enterprise. The success of that program—and the possibility that some aspects of it may yet come to timely fruition—would validate the delays. But inaction would not; unless the money, the skilled personnel, and the BL-4 laboratory suites are dedicated to this purpose, the world community is not likely to sanction further retention.

CHAPTER 6

THE MOraLITY OF EXTINCTION

Morality, religion, spirituality, superstition—call it what you will—ethical considerations have long played a leading role in humans' erratic dealings with smallpox and the variola virus. As in centuries past, our norms of collective moral philosophy inject into the ongoing global public policy debate a quiet but insistent suggestion that before proceeding toward the eradication of the remaining variola samples, we must address additional questions—obscure, ephemeral, "soft" questions, perhaps, but behind them are concerns vital for sound social choice.

GODS AND GODDESSES

It is striking—in some ways a testimony to the universality of the human experience with this disease—how many societies, widely dispersed in time and place, have associated specific deities with smallpox. These gods and goddesses have threatened people or protected them from the illness, have demanded sacrifices and tribute, and have caused populations to recoil and flee in fear. They have prescribed treatment or avoidance regimes that our modern medical insights now consider to be, variously, irrelevant, counterproductive, or insightful. In some cases, their roles have persisted for centuries.

Probably the best-known smallpox deity is the Hindu goddess Shitala mata, who fused the conflicting benevolent and horrible aspects of relief from, as well as cause of, the disease. Worshiped with mixed reverence and apprehension in India for over two millennia (although the precise date of her association with smallpox is less clear), Shitala mata is often depicted as a beautiful young woman, sitting cross-legged on a donkey, carrying a broom in one hand (for benignly brushing away the disease or savagely sweeping up nonbelievers) and an urn in the other (to dispense soothing water or to store the lethal germs for future use). Shitala mata was a prominent figure in Hindu theology, with well-attended temples devoted to her worship throughout India. The devout would pray for her to stay away from their homes, or, if she decided to visit, to rest only gently with the inhabitants. As variolation, and later vaccination, invaded Shitala mata's territory, the new technology was accommodated warily into belief systems, people concluding that medical treatment should accompany prayer, "lest the goddess not be listening or be in a pernickety and malevolent mood."[1] Her favored treatment for humans with the disease consisted of cool food and drink, enhanced by red colored powders, and fanning with leaves from the neem tree. Shitala mata seems to have risen markedly in Indian social status during the eighteenth century, evolving from a minor into a major deity; how well belief in her will survive the WHO's global elimination of her foundational disease still remains to be seen.

The corresponding Chinese goddess, T'ou-Shen Niang-Niang, can be traced back to at least the eleventh century, and she became one of the most popular objects of worship in the nineteenth century. She, too, was feared more than she was loved; it was within her power to infect a person only moderately, but she took special delight in disfiguring children with pretty faces, so on ceremonial nights Chinese children would wear ugly masks to bed, hoping to deceive the goddess into ignoring them. Temples in honor of T'ou-Shen Niang-Niang were erected all over China, and by tradition, when a person was afflicted with the disease, a close family member would be sent to take offerings to the local temple—sadly, a practice which no doubt helped the virus proliferate. Temporary shrines were also erected inside the home of a disease victim—if the acolyte recovered, the shrine was reverently burned; otherwise the goddess was cursed off the premises.

In West Africa, the Yoruba and neighboring tribes demonstrated a well-established worship of their god of smallpox, Shapona, by the seventeenth century. According to the mythology, the supreme god had delegated control over the earth to Shapona, his eldest son, who wielded smallpox as punishment when humans earned his displeasure. Each village had its own shrine to Shapona, and an annual festival in his honor was held in September—but in some quarters it was considered bad luck even to mention his name. During an epidemic, tribes were prohibited from using drums, "so that people would not congregate and be attacked by the smallpox god who may also come to dance"[2]—in effect, an administration of a quarantine. Worship in Nigeria, Togo, and Benin was led by priests now referred to as *fetisheurs,* who largely survived efforts by British colonial powers, beginning in 1907, to outlaw the population's devotion to Shapona.

In Europe, the leading illustration of this worldwide phenomenon was Saint Nicaise, the bishop of Rheims, who was killed on the steps of his church by invading Huns in A.D. 451 or 452. Saint Nicaise had recovered from smallpox a year earlier, and the Hun onslaught was shortly thereafter aborted by a widespread pestilential disease, so he became designated as the Catholic patron saint of smallpox following his canonization. Other Christian martyrs, too, were associated with salvation from smallpox: Saint Sebastian, Saint Roche, and especially Saint Barbara, who inspired such fervent worship in Luxembourg and in Soviet Georgia that the disease was sometimes identified as "Barbara-pox."[3]

Finally, the New World, too, became infused with smallpox deities, as slaves imported into northeast Brazil brought with them Yoruba-inspired traditions that merged with Roman Catholic and other expressions of faith. Known as Obaluaye ("the King of the Earth") or Omolu, the god of smallpox was represented by a dancer wrapped in straw, who performed as if doubled over in pain, imitating the suffering, trembling, and itching of a smallpox victim. In Cuba, the name of the god eventually evolved into Baba luaye, which, oddly, emerged as the title of a popular 1950s song recorded by Desi Arnaz.

In addition to these overt manifestations, religion affected smallpox in other ways, often facilitating the spread of the contagion through the community. In some instances, public ceremonies, especially funerals and the elaborate preparation of the deceased for burial, provided the occasion for multitudes to draw together, ensuring that many people would come into closer contact with the lethal virus. Other mass public ceremonies of prayer for relief from a smallpox epidemic likewise became a vehicle for accomplishing even more rapid communication of the illness. In other cases, the requirement for religious pilgrimages would promote the disease's progression to distant lands, and its periodic reimportation back home. While religion-based notions of sanitation occasionally led to traditions of isolation and quarantine of smallpox victims, more often the reverse was true, and people assembled to worship the applicable smallpox deity, unknowingly facilitating variola's further transmission.

RELIGION CONFRONTS MEDICINE

In many, if not all, communities, the emergence of modern (or premodern) medical practices for treating or preventing smallpox collided with the existing religious practices, generating severe transitional stresses with adverse reactions for both the religious and health components of social life.

Lady Montagu's introduction of variolation into England in 1721, and Cotton Mather's contemporaneous sponsorship of the practice in Boston (described in chapter 1), illustrate a social "schizophrenia": simultaneously embracing the new technology as a profound medical advance and rejecting it on religious and other grounds. Although skepticism about the concept and practice of inoculation was well deserved (it may have caused as many outbreaks as it forestalled and may ultimately have served to perpetuate smallpox in many communities), the moral outrage against the practice was particularly spirited. On both shores of the Atlantic, conservatives inveighed against variolation as (a) unchristian, since it originated in Turkey or China, or among African slaves, and was unlikely to succeed among God-fearing Caucasians; (b) unnatural, in attempting to disrupt the divine plan for human existence, in which even tragic illnesses such as smallpox were inherent, unchallengeable fixtures; and (c) blasphemous, in expressing a diabolical doubt about God's compassion for humanity, his willingness to protect his flock, and his wisdom in deciding each person's fate.

On occasion, this opposition was not merely rhetorical or abstract; it descended into physical violence against Mather and his cohorts, isolation of them from the mainstream medical community, and social ostracism. Concerted study of the novel technique, possible improvement upon it, and its propagation to those who most needed treatment were interdicted by unscientific rigidity.

Those patterns reasserted themselves early in the next century, when Jenner's vaccination revolution encountered early resistance along similar grounds. Although many religious leaders were quick to embrace the lifesaving potential of vaccination, some authorities considered it abominable to inject human beings with animal fluids such as the infective cowpox material drawn from scarified calf tissues. They fed a popular sentiment, reflected in mass market political cartoons of the era, depicting vaccinated people sprouting cow parts or growing miniature cows out of their bodies. Others contended that all disease was exclusively the province of the Lord; any human effort to prevent or minimize it—other than through the power of prayer—constituted intolerable hubris and was surely destined to damnable failure.

Those recalcitrant attitudes faded quickly with the rise of empiricism: Jenner's vaccination program demonstrably succeeded in protecting people, and throughout the Western world vaccination and religious dogma ultimately reached a mutually satisfactory modus vivendi. Even in the latter half of the twentieth century, however, the World Health Organization's global smallpox eradication campaign battled against various theocratic-based impediments as it struggled to identify, isolate, and contain smallpox outbreaks in many underdeveloped countries.

In some societies, the local priesthood resisted the WHO's vaccination publicity as the blandishments of unbelieving outsiders and decreed that a resident god of smallpox, or some other set of household deities, resolutely opposed vaccination. In many such instances, the community favored alliance with the traditional practitioners, who had served them well in many other types of crises, rather than affiliate with the "Johnny-come-lately" method of injections by outsiders. In West Africa (western Nigeria, Benin, and Togo) and in rural India, in particular, the traditional worshipers of Shapona and of Shitala mata often interfered with the vaccination movement, contending that submitting to it would displease and anger the god or goddess, incurring divine wrath in the form of even greater smallpox outbreaks, rather than protection from them.

In some instances, the practice of variolation had continued to be sustained by local priests or their associates; West African fetisheurs, in particular, posed a powerful and resistant bulwark against vaccination, for they married the indigenous religious affiliation with an economic stake in continuing to earn

fees through variolation. Often, locals under their sway would decline to identify them to WHO teams, who knew that the practice was continuing and who
experienced great difficulty in obtaining consent to proceed with their competitive technology. Some fetisheurs were also said to possess the ability to
induce the disease, as well as to prevent it, so the perceived danger of antago-
nizing them was substantial.

GENETIC ENGINEERING AND THE FRANKENSTEIN MYTH

A second, different ethical inspiration is contributed by our increasing awareness of the potential of modern genetic engineering capabilities, as outlined in
chapter 2. The prospect of creating new or genetically modified entities, for
pharmaceutical, agricultural, or weapons purposes inspires a sense of awe, even
reverence. It also carries an enormous set of unprecedented responsibilities—
first, a responsibility for safety: the danger that something in our experimentation may go awry has piqued our primal fears as in the story of Dr.
Frankenstein's monster. When people tinker with life processes we incompletely
understand, the possible adverse consequences may also exceed our compre-
hension and control.

An associated responsibility is the requirement for deeper moral inquiry.
Who are we, after all, to presume to tread into this area? By what claim of right
do we usurp such authority? Humans, of course, have always dared to challenge
nature, to shape it to our own ends. Domestication of animals and cultivation
of crops were monumental, if "unnatural" achievements. The experimentation
and exploitation of hybrid corn, cattle, and cotton through selective breeding
were usurpations of the planet's natural genetic legacy; they, too, may have
seemed dangerous, presumptuous, and foolhardy in their origins.

But genetic engineering today seems destined to stretch the limits of our
species' ken and morality to new heights. As Bernard E. Rollin puts it, modern
biological manipulation techniques constitute "evolution in the fast lane."[4] The
notion of steering DNA chains with a high degree of precision, of unwrapping
and mastering the life processes with deft expertise, carries us far beyond our
historic role on the planet. As we contemplate not only decoding but learning
to manipulate the human genome, there is reason to fear that our technological prowess may be exceeding our more slowly evolving ethical constraints.

In the case of variola, suggestions also arise from the process of decrypting, and then publishing, the complete genetic map of multiple strains of the virus. Although the viral entity is infinitely less complex than higher plants or animals, it still retains much of its mystery for us—but for how long? Could scientists armed with the detailed map and with exquisite gene splicing techniques create "from scratch" an exact replica of variola? If so, would it function as its "parent" model did, with all the processes of infection, growth, and reproduction? And in the process, would humans then be able to claim a truly god-like capability to breathe "life" onto our planet?

THE ETHICS OF EXTINCTION

A set of equally profound and perplexing questions awaits us as we contemplate humanity's role at the opposite end of the life cycle: the termination, rather than the creation, of a species. Once again, much of the novel and troubling activity has a traditional, unproblematic base: species become extinct all the time, for a wide variety of reasons. As outlined in chapter 4, throughout the earth's history, the only constant in biology has been change: climatic conditions, natural selection, and pure happenstance have driven countless forms of plant and animal life out of existence. Human beings have had little to do with the bulk of these species and their extinctions, for better or worse, which have proceeded largely unnoticed and unlamented. In other cases, people have been an agent of extermination, either directly (e.g., via overhunting) or indirectly (e.g., via destruction of a vital habitat).

At this point in our social and ethical evolution, it may be appropriate to consider three levels of participation, or roles, that humans might have in an extinction morality play: (a) *causing* the extermination of a species; (b) being *conscious* about the part we are playing; and (c) deciding *deliberately* to make it happen, as a desired outcome.

For much of our prehistoric experience on earth, humans probably contributed little to the extermination process. There were so few people, and their technology was so primitive, that their collective impact upon the planet's flora and fauna was limited. Over time, people came, collectively, to fulfill the first of those differentiated roles with increasing frequency. In greater numbers and with larger "footprints," we tampered with sensitive ecological balances, knowing or caring little what decisions we were implicitly making for other fragile entities. We caused their deaths, clumsily or stupidly, with ignorance our only defense.

Within the last century or two, we have occasionally elevated our sights, to achieve the second level noted above, becoming collectively conscious of our role in the precipitous decline of, for example, dodo birds or passenger pigeons. Sometimes we were indifferent to the fact, but sometimes we opted to arrest the trend, protecting at least some handfuls of favored species from the dustbin of history. With our current levels of modern insight and scientific technique, we are now more often aware of our role in unsettling some of these ecological equilibriums and more deft at avoiding the worst consequences.

It is not clear which, if either, of these two postures is morally superior: is it preferable to be an ignorant blunderer, unthinkingly wreaking havoc upon other creatures, or is it in any way better to be aware of the harsh consequences of one's deeds but regularly proceed forward nonetheless, in pursuit of chosen human goals, despite their costs to other species?

In any event, the variola question now brings humankind, for the first time, to the precipice of the third level, where we might *deliberately* decide to terminate an entire species. This is another monumental step, worthy of our collective pause. As Jonathan Schell observed in the context of nuclear war, and the threat it poses to survival of the human race, there is, analytically, a critical distinction between the death of an individual and the extermination of a species. He asks us to imagine two separate situations: one in which many people—millions, or even billions, of our species—are somehow suddenly killed, but the planet's essential life-sustaining processes and components that our kind depends on are sustained, and our race is able, in time, to recover, to continue fruitful breeding, and to repopulate. The second hypothetical situation would be one in which a mysterious force suddenly rendered all human beings irreversibly sterile: no current lives would be taken, no physical pain inflicted, but there would be no future generations, and as the existing population declined, the earth would lose the last vestiges of humanity.[5]

Each of these bizarre scenarios would constitute an unthinkable tragedy, and it is not Schell's thesis to argue that either is "worse" than the other—just that they are distinct and that a cataclysmic nuclear war, and the prolonged, sun-light-blocking nuclear winter that might follow it, would run the risk of incurring, in sequence, the worst versions of each model.

No one would hint that the elimination of the last variola samples is an event with the same moral consequence as nuclear holocaust, but the two cases do share the finality, the irreversibility of extinction. Making a permanent mark on our planet—and deciding to do so consciously and deliberately—is the most powerful sort of statement we humans could make about our position in earth's environment, and it should be rife with ethical inhibitions.

There is, to be sure, an offsetting moral argument of an essential sort: self-preservation. The variola virus has for three or four millennia been one of the most pernicious, stubborn killers of humans. The record of pain and suffering provides justification for a massive social response and surely merits extreme measures to contain the threat and to snuff out its future dangers to our progeny. Only by final elimination can we be certain that variola will not somehow reemerge to jeopardize our descendants in the same way it terrified our ancestors.

In that vein, we have already, without yielding to any ethical inhibitions, removed all traces of the virus from the active biosphere. We struggled mightily—heroically—against this foe, destroying as many exemplars as possible and confining the few lingering remnants to secure isolation. If it is proper—and it must be—for humans to act so stridently in this manner, to extirpate this creature from its only viable niche in nature, why would it be any less moral for us to consign the final hardy remnants to an autoclave? Moreover, in pursuing the ethical strain of the argument too far, we might lose sight of what is really at stake within the realm of endangered species. It seems odd for people to spend much time deliberating over retention or destruction of variola when there are many other, more clear-cut cases of endangered species crying out for protection. If we somehow allow ourselves to be diverted even momentarily from the pressing needs for husbanding our most vital plant and animal neighbors, it would be a serious misallocation of our resources and our compassion.

A concluding observation about the unusual nature of this extermination/preservation issue: Ordinarily, questions of this sort resolve themselves into struggles over resources. People ask, "Is it really worth it to save species X, when doing so would mean foregoing (or resiting, or paying more for) a planned highway, shopping mall, or housing subdivision?" While it is often complex to evaluate in monetary terms the value of the jeopardized species, the price for saving it can be calculated (albeit routinely exaggerated for effect) and can be substantial.

In the case of variola, however, it's not principally a question of opportunity costs that weigh against preservation: The price for sustaining the virus is low: the trivial increment of electricity for the freezers, the marginal wages of the security guards, and other provisions are minimal. The danger that the virus might escape is important, of course, and it appears that most people have blind spots when it comes to evaluating outcomes that are unlikely to occur but that would be disastrous if they did eventuate. Still, most of our collective experience, much of the literature on species preservation, and a great deal of the litigation in the field are largely inapplicable here: the values being balanced in the case of variola are not principally financial, and that component of public policy decision making is virtually removed from the ethical dimension of our story.

THE SYMBOLISM OF ERADICATION

What message do we send, to ourselves and to our posterity, by eradicating or by preserving variola? What does this extermination represent; what does it say about our species, our self-perceptions, and our place within nature?

There is, first, a powerful positive symbolism in marking humanity's final victory over smallpox—a triumphant culmination of the ancient battle, to be capped with a guarantee that the foe can never return. Nothing else could so vividly represent our complete success in this millennial battle against a horrific, disgusting scourge. Nothing else could so boldly convey the resolute unanimity and finality that the world has brought to this unprecedented question. As one Russian smallpox expert puts it, if the planet's epochal struggle against variola were to end without total eradication, "it would be as if a piece of music were to end before the final note was struck."[6]

And the WHO smallpox eradication campaign was one of our species' finest moments, uniting peoples of the world; allowing them to momentarily set aside their political, military, and economic battles; inspiring them to pool political will, inventiveness, technology, capital, and commitment to a common good. The event richly deserves to be celebrated, remembered, and symbolically preserved. The symbolic value of culminating the planetary struggle against smallpox may, in fact, prove to be the strongest point in favor of the virus's eradication. Because it would be such an unprecedented event, a departure from our otherwise noble (if relatively newfound) instincts to respect and preserve species, it would notify the world that something very unusual has occurred. The symbolism of variola eradication—decades after smallpox eradication— would communicate to everyone the value we place upon this human accomplishment, ensure that the triumph is not undone by future incompetence or malevolence, and perpetuate for our successors the notion that a heroic step of indelible proportions has been recorded.

A commitment to the eradication of variola could also contribute to a deepening global sense that some forms of combat, biological weapons in particular, are wholly out of bounds for civilized societies. In the words of D. A. Henderson, we need to "create a moral climate where smallpox is considered too morally reprehensible to be used as a weapon."[7] Abolition would make any retained variola, in any covert laboratory or military facility, prima facie illegal and by extension its possessors to be rogues, enemies of all people.

As with most moral argumentation, this point of symbolism admits of counterarguments. It might be asserted that the greater symbolic value would be to preserve the virus in vitro, to demonstrate, if not our compassion for this undeserving foe, at least our appreciation that even a loathsome little creature like variola may have a place in nature's grand scheme. In fact, perhaps the best way to memorialize humanity's victory would be through mercy: to sustain the frozen virus samples forever, as an artifact of the heroic struggle. By this reasoning, perhaps we should make (denatured fragments of) the virus available for public display; people appreciate the opportunity to gawk at the accoutrements of great evil: we queue up for museum exhibitions of Nazi memorabilia and wax impressions of mass murderers. We take care to preserve samples of Civil War detritus and retired cold war ICBMs. We seem to believe that the public can be educated, impressed, and entertained by viewing these relics or simply by knowing that these once dangerous reminders of our common legacy still exist. Perhaps an even greater symbolic statement of our mastery over smallpox would be demonstrated not by destroying the last exemplars of the variola virus but by so thoroughly taming them that we can confidently retain them as a collective reminder of how far we have progressed together.

Finally, the symbolism of deliberate extinction of any species, including a lowly virus, implicates the most fundamental notions of humankind's interactions with nature throughout the eons. As David Ehrenfeld writes, "This non-humanistic value of communities and species is the simplest of all to state: they should be conserved because they exist and because this existence is itself but the present expression of a continuing historical process of immense antiquity and majesty. Long-standing existence in Nature is deemed to carry with it the unimpeachable right to continued existence."[8] According to this basic normative principle, preservation of the "existence value" of variola—provided it could be accomplished safely—is simply the right thing to do, in expressing, both symbolically and realistically, respect for the world around us.

FACTORS OBSCURING MORAL JUDGMENTS

The difficulty in obtaining a perspective allowing clear ethical judgments in this complicated area is already apparent. This section sketches three additional factors that can obscure our collective insights and that inevitably touch, but should not control, our moral reasoning about variola.

First, we must deal with the debate over whether the virus is considered "alive." As elaborated in chapter 2, most biologists would maintain that a creature so dependent on other beings for the basic functions of life—a virus cannot move, grow, or reproduce without commandeering the assistance from an involuntary host—does not fit within the traditional confines of living things. Even for many nonscientists, there is a dividing line between creatures we conceptualize as being alive and for which we must sustain some special regard, and entities, such as viruses, that do not properly rise to that level.

From this perspective, the "fate" of variola is no more a proper subject of human concern, compassion, or ethical consideration than would be the fate of some inanimate machine or inert collection of random chemicals. We should feel no more reluctance or hesitance in destroying it than we do when we extract carcinogenic chemicals from our foods or pollutants from our smokestacks, or when we abandon obsolete automobiles or computers to the junkyard—all are just chemical compounds, elaborately arranged, not living entities.

Along these lines, if we pursue the structure of the Biological Weapons Convention, discussed in chapter 3, we note that the basic prohibitions of its article 1 identify three distinct categories of regulated substances: (1) "microbial or other biological agents" (the bacterium, virus, and so on, that causes a disease); (2) "toxins whatever their origin or method of production" (i.e., nonliving substances produced by living entities that injure or kill without reproducing themselves or causing a disease); and (3) "weapons, equipment or means of delivery designed to use such agents or toxins" (the bombs, canisters, spray devices, and the like intended to contain, transport, and disseminate the noxious substances).[9] Clearly the latter two categories—toxins and delivery systems—are nonliving and would not properly be the subject of the same type of human compassion and moral philosophy we reserve for living things. By that same logic, we could categorize a virus as closer to an inert set of molecules, more like a delivery system than like a living being. If so, we could discard variola with no more ethical qualms than we would have in crushing or burning the missiles or aerosol generators connected with it.

This analysis, however powerful, overlooks two complications. First, the dividing line, both in biology and ethics, between living and nonliving entities, is not so clear-cut. The defining characteristics of life are inevitably at least somewhat fuzzy around the extreme edges, as the wonders of our natural world sometimes defy the neat categorizing schemes invented by human minds. Even a virus displays some of the characteristics of life and is a biological entity, a life form, a proper subject of life sciences investigation. A virus does not appear to be markedly different, at least not in the sense that renders moral judgment unnecessary, from creatures one step on the other side of the constructed life/nonlife dividing line. Are bacteria, rickettsia, and fungi so much more advanced or different in chemistry, function, and position in the environment that they are dramatically more suitable subjects for human ethical contemplation? A virus, in short, is different from an inert molecule; it is not of the same stature as a chemical or toxin. At the least, the subtle differences between the various entities and their respective niches in the biological hierarchy do not allow us to draw rigid ethical distinctions between creatures located at nearly contiguous points on the continuum.

Supporting this argument is the contention that even if a virus is regarded as "non-living," as being stuck on the disfavored side of the great biological demarcation, that conclusion does not free us from all ethical consideration of it. Some clearly nonliving, nonbiological, insentient, inert entities are properly the subject of human ethical evaluation. Monumental natural phenomena (the Grand Canyon, the Appalachian Mountains), historically significant man-made works (the Great Wall of China, the Eiffel Tower), and creations that mix both (rocks brought back from the moon, boulders arranged at Stonehenge) are not "biological," yet there would be some strong ethical content, going beyond simple sentimentality, to any decision to destroy or alter them. Consideration for future generations of humans, for preserving the historic and natural splendor of our planet, would mandate that we preserve them, or at least think about the moral implications of any decision to eliminate them. Even nonliving "things" can earn the right to be taken seriously, to be the subject of moral judgment going beyond simple sentimentality. Even if the subject of the inquiry—such as the variola virus—is not alive in the traditional sense, we still have an unavoidable obligation to step carefully through the moral minefield in deciding its fate.

The second obscuring factor arises from the question of whether human society still has a "use" for this particular virus. As noted in chapter 2, humans might discern, or develop, a utility in further medical research on this creature, following Ovid's advice that "we can learn even from our enemies."[10] As mentioned earlier, such developments might include a new smallpox vaccine with fewer side effects and contraindications; improved antiviral medications; and more generalized insights into the human immune system and the principles of viral infectivity.

And we should also be appropriately modest about our ability to predict *future* needs or uses for a unique creature like variola. Who knows what applications unborn generations might find for this odd packaging of DNA, as science expands in unforeseen directions in distant decades? Our repeated inability to date to predict the historical evolutions and revolutions of science should make us wary about blanket projections of what our progeny might find useful or even essential some day. The "flip side" of our apprehension over the possible unforeseen negative consequences of ambitious activities such as genetic engineering would be our hope that there could be currently unappreciated future advantages to leaving some things just the way they are.

But whether variola still has, or might one day have, a value for people cannot be the sole determinant of its fate. We cannot ethically demand that all creatures on the planet "earn" their right to survival by demonstrating that they are "useful" to human beings. Even the most homocentric perspectives would not focus exclusively upon that test for extinction, even for the most execrable life-forms.

There has long been something of a debate among environmentalists, religious authorities, and others about whether we should protect the natural environment: (a) in order to protect people, by preserving the values and virtues that are found only in the wild, or (b) for its own sake. We need not attempt to resolve that conundrum here; it is sufficient to conclude that utility is not the exclusive or even the dominating force in moral inquiries about species preservation. There is simply more to it than that.

Religious teachings amplify the point. While most traditions are sometimes equivocal about humans' permission (or even requirement) to master, subdue, and exploit the earth, there is also a strong stream of modern sectarian philosophy demanding respect for nature, living in harmony with God's creation and zealously safeguarding the planet for our successors. Diverse religious literature abounds with phrases about all living creatures being mankind's companions and about our responsibility for generous stewardship of the divine dominion—a mandate having little to do with notions of utility. So whether we have a scientific need to retain these remnants of the variola virus, we may still properly feel a desire, or even an obligation, not to expunge it from the planet.

The third impediment to moral judgment about the eradication question is reflected in the analogies that pervade the literature. The most common, seemingly irresistible, journalistic metaphors about variola liken the virus to a criminal prisoner (usually one convicted of mass murder), incarcerated on death row, invulnerable to any rehabilitation efforts, while the international authorities debate whether to grant yet another stay of execution. A similarly hardy rhetoric borrows from the vocabulary of military campaigns, calling the viral samples "prisoners of war," who remain captive years after the glorious combat has been concluded. Pursuing that rhetoric, it is easy to justify the permanent confinement of variola, locking it forever in frozen test tubes, with only the occasional forays for testing or experimentation. Smallpox was, after all, a vile disease, a devastating threat to mankind—it could be seen as the viral equivalent of *Silence of the Lambs*'s evil Hannibal Lecter—and the eradication campaign against it was a brilliant, wondrous success. Self-preservation is, of course, a first priority for the human race, so the permanent "solitary confinement" or eventual "capital punishment" of the incorrigible virus seems morally justified.

Yet, these simple analogies do not fully ring true, and they even suggest countervailing points that carry the analysis in odd and contradictory directions. Even prisoners, after all, have certain rights. What due process protections should be applied in the case of variola? What substantive standards should define the "crime" for which the virus's liberty and life may be revoked? What would count as cruel and unusual punishment in this first-ever application of a species' capital punishment? What does it mean for a microscopic creature to be guilty of a criminal act, when it is incapable of conscious or deliberate action, and is only fulfilling the role that nature prescribed for it?

Thirty years ago, Christopher Stone's pathbreaking (and still controversial) suggestion that trees and other insensate entities might have legal "standing"—the ability to litigate cases in their own names and to receive financial or other remedies to be applied for their own benefit—was either disconcerting or mildly amusing to the legal system.[11] Yet, as he argues, other nonhuman creations (corporations, partnerships, estates) have long enjoyed legal "personality"—although at one time, the notion that such fictional beings could sue and be sued, own property, receive money, and act in their own capacities was regarded as similarly bizarre and untenable. He posits that it makes equally good sense to allow a dog to sue (via a *guardian ad litem* of some sort) for cruelty inflicted upon it; for a lake to litigate over pollution dumped into it; or for a species to claim directly in court the right to preservation—instead of continuing to rely upon the strained notions of "injury in fact" to nearby human beings and organizations who must contort the reality in order to claim some legally sufficient causal link to the offending action.

If it is imaginable that a river valley, through suitable human representatives, could become legally competent to assert its own rights to cleanliness or physical integrity, could it likewise be possible for the variola virus to raise a cognizable claim to a "liberty" interest in avoiding permanent incarceration, or, with greater force, in avoiding death and species extermination? If we have a commitment to "humane" treatment of animals, does that imply that even microscopic entities might have a defensible stake in "rights" that could be vindicated in court and that have to be assessed according to principled legal standards, rather than through the ad hoc justice dispensed via the WHO's political multilateral voting procedures?

These are hard questions—and they get harder the more deeply one thinks about them. But resolution is not materially aided, I submit, by adopting the metaphors of criminal justice. The loose talk about capital punishment for variola might be helpful in arresting our attention, in compelling us to pause and think more deeply about where our natural instincts might otherwise automatically lead us. But the analogies can carry us only so far into moral inquiries; the difficult ethical analysis must proceed on its own unique terms in this unprecedented venue.

THE PRECEDENTIAL IMPACT

As has been repeatedly noted, there has never been anything like the pending variola decision, but other iterations of this thorny problem lie not far into our future. While we cannot be certain what unfortunate little creature will be the next on the WHO chopping block, we can be confident (or apprehensive) that something will be jeopardized, and perhaps not long from now, so that our evolving moral judgments will be put to the test repeatedly within this generation's life span.

One likely candidate is polio. This terrible disease, like smallpox, has crippled and killed humans for centuries. Like smallpox, it is caused by a virus, and, once again, it is a rather unusual virus in that it infects only human beings, without a stable animal or other reservoir, so global eradication is a feasible objective. And the campaign against the disease has registered enormous successes: already polio is essentially absent from the Western Hemisphere, the World Health Organization has formally adopted the goal of complete planetary eradication, and hundreds of millions of dollars have been devoted to the effort.

While success can never be guaranteed, within a few years, the polio virus may exist only in a small number of well-guarded and tightly regulated national laboratories. The analysis of whether, at that time, to proceed with polio's final eradication will, perhaps, draw upon many of the same dimensions assessed in this book, but surely there will be important variations, too. Polio, for example, has never been a plausible candidate for use as a biological weapon—for all the horror it causes, it is too slow-acting for military or terrorist purposes.

Who knows what diseases will then fall in humankind's relentless progression against suffering? We might tackle guinea worm fever next, or malaria, or measles. Those and other noxious impairments are caused by a set of viruses, bacteria, and parasites that have only grudgingly yielded to human control, but perhaps greater success is on the horizon. There can be, at this point, no timetable for concluding, or even initiating, ambitious global campaigns for many illnesses, but if one adopts an outlook measured in decades, it is fully predictable that other creatures, and not just nonliving viruses, will be brought to the stage of potential eradication.

At that point, perhaps, our sense of communal ethics—along with our judgments about the medical, biological, environmental, and other dimensions of the issue—will be sufficiently refined to allow the planet to draw upon mature moral reflection, as well as upon whatever precedent we create in the early twenty-first century. It should not be too much to hope that our sense of social ethics—as well as our technology—can evolve and mature over time (probably just not quite as rapidly).

Procedural as well as substantive aspects of ethical justice will have to be addressed: Will we appoint some sort of international guardian or ombudsman for the polio virus, to advocate on its behalf? Should there at least be court-appointed legal counsel in instances of litigation or similar formal proceedings? Will we have some sort of notice-and-comment proceeding for the parasitic worm responsible for dracunculiasis, through which all voices can be heard to express opinions regarding what is likely to be another intricate choice between continued retention in laboratories and total eradication? Will we be driven, somehow, to feel empathy for the microorganism that causes bubonic plague— and would that be a sign of greater moral sensitivity in the human species or an indicator of effete, misplaced emotionalism? Who would be the relevant populations to participate in these momentous deliberations—all people on the planet, or just citizens of the countries that still happened to retain stocks of the relevant bug? Is it to be decided by scientific experts, international bureaucrats, or global plebiscite?

CONCLUSION

Variola genuinely presents a case of global "first impression," and humans will obtain little direct guidance from textbooks on moral philosophy. This first brush with deliberate extermination of a species is an occasion of historic proportions, laden with powerful symbolism—one way or the other—about who we human beings are and what we assert as our position within our cosmos.

Variola, to be sure, makes an odd poster child for biodiversity, preservation of life-forms, or cross-species empathy. Yet, sometimes, we have to take our moments of moral judgment where we find them, and this one is now inescapable. As a matter of sheer pragmatism, we cannot dodge the occasion for confronting deep truth.

One way to approach the issue, only partially pushing it into the future, would be to insert a form of burden of proof. That is, one might surmise that a version of the precautionary principle should be applied: when in doubt, avoid irreversible steps. (By analogy, many computer programs initialize their default settings in such a manner that if the user makes a mistake, or unthinkingly proceeds past warning signs, the least consequential alternative will be automatically selected, and the user must deliberately opt for any of the more powerful outcomes.) In this fashion, the burden of proof would be on those who advocate destruction; if they were unable to build a completely satisfactory case, then the entity (variola in this case, something else tomorrow) would be preserved at least temporarily, until the next occasion for review arose.

Under that logic, the ethical question changes from "What should we do with the last samples of the virus?" into the more judgmental "By what right do we destroy it?" There may be a sufficient moral basis for destroying variola, today or at some point in the future, but it would have to be comprehensively and publicly proffered. As of today, the ethical doubts persist.

Another implication of the ethical question is the line drawing or slippery slope conundrum: if it is morally permissible to destroy all variola, what other creatures could likewise be exterminated? Are all viruses vulnerable, as a class? Or only those that cause dread diseases? What about bacteria and other microscopic organisms? What about benign or positively useful bacteria? As we proceed to multicelled parasitic creatures, and then plants, insects, and lower animals, at what point do our collective moral judgments kick in? We would not intentionally destroy a familiar animal species—at least not in situations where the cost of retention was so low. But are our moral thermometers sufficiently sensitive to identify salient, reliable distinctions among biological formats?

One approach to the "bottom line," ethically speaking, may be to return to the notion of rights. If a creature such as the variola virus can have a claim to any rights, what would they be, and how strong would they be? (Recall that within the realm of ethics, as well as law, merely identifying and holding a right of some sort is far from the end of the story; such rights often come into conflict, and judges and moral authorities must assess their relative strengths and their applicability to any particular situation.) Two hypothetical rights might appear here: a right to liberty (i.e., to existence "in the wild," outside the frozen laboratory test tubes) and a right to survival (i.e., to sustenance as a species).

The liberty right—comparable to a person's freedom of movement, freedom from incarceration, and so on—is ordinarily very powerful. We instinctively hesitate to interfere with a liberty claim, absent the greatest provocation. But in the case of variola, there is such a provocation: the threat that the virus inherently carries for all humans. Under those circumstances—an overwhelming Us versus Them situation—the self-preservation interest of humans clearly outweighs the proposed liberty rights of the virus, and permanent relegation to the laboratory deep freeze is appropriate.

The survival right, however, might be balanced differently. Survival of the species is perhaps the most basic, most important "right" that any entity can hold. Even in the case of an entity such as a virus, considered by many to be nonliving, if we extend recognition to any of its possible claims of right, this would one be the most enduring and the hardest to outweigh.

What interest of humans would then trump variola's "right" to sheer existence? It might not take a strong human interest to overcome this most basic viral right, but it would take something—and human self-preservation has already been taken into account (except, perhaps, for the exceedingly low, but not zero, probability of a theft, escape, or accidental release from a storage laboratory).

Although the answers to those questions are hard to come by, we must struggle to address them. The bottom-line danger, drawn from an ethical dimension, is that technology and the monumental success of the smallpox eradication campaign have brought humanity to a situation where our careening power has outstripped our more slowly evolving moral education. We certainly have the ability to extinguish variola and other species; we just cannot yet be clear whether we have the moral authority to do so, or the wisdom to think with clarity about the opportunity.

CHAPTER 7

THE case for extermination

It is now time to put it all together. This chapter and the next meld the lessons of the prior chapters by assembling the best possible case *for* promptly destroying the last smallpox virus samples (here), and the strongest array of arguments *against* that policy (chapter 8). The effort is to integrate, in the context of irreversible planetary decision making, the insights gained from the dimensions of medicine, biology, military science, environmentalism, international organizations, and ethics.[1]

As is traditional with courtroom decorum, the moving party, the one who seeks to disturb the status quo, presents its case first. Accordingly, this chapter marshals five arguments in favor of destroying the last variola; each is accompanied by a rebuttal.

ARGUMENT 1: *It costs money to continue to store and work on this stuff.* The first argument is simple, direct, and incontrovertible. Ongoing storage and processing of variola stockpiles consume resources that could be saved or reallocated to other purposes. The 450 vials in Atlanta and the 120 in Novosibirsk occupy space in the laboratory freezers, space that is increasingly at a premium as those facilities continue or expand their other enterprises.

It is difficult to calculate precisely the marginal cost of permanent retention of the variola stocks. However, any assessment should consider a fair pro rata allocation of the overall institutional expenditures for space, electrical energy, laboratory equipment, and security. Together, those costs would not be negligible.

In Russia, especially, adequate, secure laboratory space is notoriously scarce—as evidenced by the necessity, in 1994, of suddenly transporting the variola inventory from the Ivanovsky Institute in Moscow, where it could not be sufficiently protected. The world shudders at the fact that highly sensitive materials—the key ingredients for nuclear, chemical, and other weapons of mass destruction—are routinely unsafeguarded in Russia. One commentator has observed that "even potatoes are protected better," and the lack of hard currency has impeded efforts to build new, stronger facilities or to upgrade and expand existing units. Where savings can be effectuated such as by eliminating unnecessary biological warfare components from the stockpiles, the opportunity should not be squandered.

Carrying this argument one step further, the costs of progressing from passive storage of infectious variola materials to active research on them, are substantial. It is, once again, hard to put an accurate price tag on such an open-ended, ill-defined enterprise, but the goals of the program are so ambitious that the budget must be appreciable. Moreover, the "opportunity costs" of any such effort are especially daunting—given the shortage of BL-4 facilities and the small number of expert virologists available to undertake the inquiries, we should be keenly aware of the displacement that occurs when smallpox research usurps the possibility of devoting those resources to other pressing needs, from AIDS to the Ebola virus to the West Nile virus.

REBUTTAL 1:   The financial price for retaining the existing smallpox stocks is trivial. Compressed into a modest collection of vials, they require no maintenance, no "care and feeding," only virtually costless passive monitoring. They occupy a small amount of freezer space, consuming a minimal amount of refrigeration energy.

Moreover, the *marginal* cost to the facility is close to nil. With or without these variola samples, the Centers for Disease Control and Prevention in Atlanta and the Research Center of Virology and Biotechnology in Novosibirsk will continue their existing operations essentially unchanged. They could not truly save much freezer space, personnel, or other costs. The infrastructure is already in place, and smallpox-related activities are such a small part of the operation that the bottom line is impervious to their coming or going. Because of all the *other*, even more noxious, substances that will continue to be housed there, the laboratories will have to sustain all the elaborate and costly BL-4 facilities into the indefinite future. Therefore, no security guards could be discharged, no electronic monitoring systems could be relaxed, even if variola instantly went the way of the dodo.

Moreover, any valid assessment of the "costs" of the further retention and examination of the variola inventory must in fairness look at the "benefit" side of the ledger, too. If our ongoing research program does yield new insights into virology, human immunology, and the like, the long-term gains for human health and well-being could be enormous. While that upside potential is admittedly speculative, it is certainly plausible and could come to swamp the costs we now incur.

To the extent that costs are a consideration, it is probably true that the world has already spent more on *studies* of the variola elimination question (via WHO committees and conferences, research papers, and books such as this one) than could possibly be saved by eliminating the virus.

ARGUMENT 2: *Continued storage incurs an inherent risk that the virus might escape by accident or design, potentially incurring enormous social dangers and costs.* There are a great many all-too-plausible "scare scenarios" in which variola returns to the unprotected world. Natural catastrophes or human accidents, ranging from earthquakes to plane crashes to building fires cannot be entirely discounted. Atlanta, Georgia, for example, is buffeted by severe storms as regularly as any other area: Fulton County has been declared a presidential disaster area on five occasions since 1990, following devastating collisions with Hurricane Opal (1995), Tropical Storm Alberto (1994), and others. Despite efforts to make the CDC facilities as physically sound as possible, and to locate the most sensitive materials in the most impregnable corridors of the building, there is some (admittedly low) level of risk that cannot be totally removed: no building can withstand the power of nature's worst furies.

Negligence or recklessness by key personnel is a permanent danger, too. In any industry, there is a statistical probability of errors and accidents, even profound mishaps. Sound training and personnel practices attempt to reduce this incidence to a tolerably low level, but it is hubris to suggest that catastrophes such as those at Three Mile Island, Chernobyl, or Bhopal could never recur.

Deliberately hostile human intervention, as well as those unintentional accidents, must also be factored into the security equation. Terrorists could attack a laboratory; if sufficiently armed, trained, and disciplined, they would have some nonzero probability of successfully "liberating" disease agents that could serve their ends. One need not be a Nostradamus to foresee, in the aftermath of the incidents at the World Trade Center, the Oklahoma City federal building, and the Tokyo subway, the possibility of ambitious, well-financed, and possibly suicidal zealots.

More insidiously, hostile foreign governments, or perhaps organized (or even disorganized) crime elements, could attempt to bribe impoverished or disgruntled laboratory employees, providing access to infectious materials that might command a lofty price on the international black market. The Aldrich Ames and Robert Hanssen espionage cases demonstrate that even the innermost circles of the CIA and the FBI are susceptible to financial inducements; every other institution must have its weak points, too.

There is already ample evidence of these dangers emerging inside modern Russia: cadres of formerly elite military officials, weapons experts, and other government personnel are now reduced in status and income, perhaps rendering them vulnerable to bribes and other blandishments. Almost anything is now available on the Russian black market—guns, chemicals, sensitive technology; as long as those conditions prevail, variola cannot be considered absolutely secure.

Moreover, these alternative scenarios cannot be dismissed as fictionalized nightmares: some of them have happened. Even Louis Pasteur's laboratory was victimized by accidents that spread rabies while he was attempting to develop a viral vaccine. More recently, twice during the 1970s, variola was accidentally released from laboratories in England, infecting and killing unsuspecting victims. In retrospect, we can identify inadequate safety precautions in both those London and the Birmingham tragedies, and the current standards far surpass those that were applicable at the time. Yet, this type of hindsight is always 100 percent successful, and those facilities were, in their day, considered reasonably secure for this hazardous activity. Can we afford to be any more self-congratulatory about laboratory stringency today?

American military operations have experienced their share of mishaps, too. Chemical weapons leaking from the Dugway testing facility in Utah in 1968 killed thousands of sheep; the Army's secret testing of CBW simulants in U.S. cities in the 1950s and 1960s exposed thousands of people to unknown risks; and the danger that spies might steal or purchase secrets is not confined to any one society. In 1997 an American fighter pilot, perhaps distraught over romantic failures or other stresses, flew away with his A-10 fighter, leaving a training mission in Arizona and slipping off the radar screen for hours, in a fully armed aircraft capable of massive combat. If a single deranged pilot can make off with a $9 million vehicle on a suicide rampage, what could happen with a simple test tube?[2]

In addition, we must not lose sight of the fact that the world of smallpox and public health has changed in other significant ways since the 1970s—some of which would make a potential "variola excursion" more tragic than previously. First, a dwindling percentage of humans now have reliable immunity. Few people have been vaccinated in the past few decades—the United States suspended routine antismallpox injections for the civilian population in the early 1970s and now has well over 100 million citizens who have never been vaccinated. For most of those vaccinated as young children, the passage of time has rendered the original treatment largely ineffective. (Those vaccinations probably conferred full protection for perhaps ten years.) The world today has few survivors of smallpox; since the disease has been thankfully removed from the inventory of human pestilence for over two decades, there remain few people who acquired the disease, outlasted it, and thereby achieved lifetime immunity.

In short, the human population now has lost most of the "herd immunity" that limited the virulence of smallpox epidemics. In earlier centuries, a smallpox outbreak, as devastating as it was, knew natural bounds—once variola had ravaged the unprotected population of an area, it would butt up against the residual group that had survived previous attacks, and the virus would run out of fresh victims. Today, however, that protection is largely gone, and the entire globe is in a situation more nearly reminiscent of that of Native Americans during the sixteenth and seventeenth centuries. Lacking any prior exposure to variola, whole tribes were eradicated when the virus was first set upon them. The comparable type of exposure today could therefore far exceed the toll exacted by the 1979 Sverdlovsk anthrax outbreak—the most recent escapade with a released BW agent.

A subsidiary point here is that our domestic and international public health system—which in general makes the global health situation radically better than that of prior centuries—is no longer honed to a great sensitivity regarding variola. Generations of doctors and nurses have never seen a case of smallpox; hospitals have no current experience with handling the disease. Cases might not be immediately recognized and identified, for no one has been called upon to make this diagnosis for over twenty years. Confirming the symptoms of smallpox and initiating appropriate treatment and quarantine procedures are therefore no longer practiced routines. While the U.S. system could probably be mobilized and trained relatively quickly to generate a suitable medical response to an outbreak, the resources elsewhere might not be so available.

Added to these conceivable adverse events is the possibility of a mutation of variola. The virus has apparently undergone a number of transformations in its devastating career, and it is somehow related to a whole family of other disease agents, most of which are similar but less noxious to humans. Monkey pox in Central Africa today seems to be demonstrating this sort of capacity for hostile mutation, becoming a more deadly scourge than before. How could we be confident that these poxvirus transformations will not occur again in the future and perhaps this time in the direction of creating an even more deadly variant of the germ? As long as variola is sustained, and as long as the possibility—however remote—exists that it might escape and mutate, the dangers cannot truly be confined to the realm of lurid science fiction.

REBUTTAL 2: These dangers are greatly exaggerated; the probability of any realistic virus escape scenario is vanishingly small. The WHO has recently surveyed the two collaborating centers and found them adequate to the challenge of safe and secure storage. Of course, nothing in life can be absolutely certain, and if additional safety procedures or equipment can be identified, developed, and implemented, to further reduce the risk of accidental or deliberate leakage, those steps may be welcomed as incremental supplements to an already-tight security apparatus. In particular, if more could be done to strengthen the

Russian protective protocols, that may well be a suitable expenditure of money, including American aid funds.

But it is also noteworthy that the imagined dangers would be only slightly abated, even if all traces of variola were immediately destroyed. That is, the facilities that currently hold smallpox residues also house samples of many other, equally deadly substances. Those agents—viruses, bacteria, rickettsias, and so on, that cause or carry many of the worst diseases known to humans—will linger, regardless of the outcome of the current smallpox debate. Accordingly, hurricanes, earthquakes, and plane crashes could still unleash pestilence; terrorists could still seize biological warfare agents; organized crime could still bribe or blackmail impoverished employees to turn over access to dangerous substances. Technology, money, and concerted effort might help mitigate those dangers, but elimination of any one pathogen, such as variola, at a time when so many other, equally hostile substances will remain in the laboratory inventory, would not appreciably alter the odds or the potential outcomes.

Moreover, we should not gainsay that the world does have the capacity to respond even to these types of dire emergencies. The United States and the WHO have continued to stockpile millions of doses of vaccinia virus—as well as the feedstocks capable of producing more vaccine, should the need emerge—and the production of hundreds of millions of additional doses is being arranged with newfound urgency. Those inventories would be maintained indefinitely, regardless of what is done with variola. Likewise, the technology for swiftly administering protection through mass injections has not eroded or been forgotten—indeed, it has been improved. On the human and organizational level, we know how to deal with smallpox outbreaks—the world proved that conclusively during the 1970s—and we should be able to interdict a modern plague relatively rapidly. Again, there can be no guarantees, but variola, if somehow released from captivity, would never again be allowed to run endlessly amok.

ARGUMENT 3: *There is a powerful affirmative symbolism for all humankind in finally and thoroughly ridding the planet of this despicable disease agent.* Symbolism is important, especially in matters of public policy debate. One aspect of this symbolism arises from the opportunity for people to demonstrate that, through concerted, self-conscious action, our species can exert a powerful, positive impact upon the natural environment. Much of our interaction with the biosphere is profoundly negative and selfish: we consume irreplaceable resources at a frightening rate; we pollute the ecosystems that we and other species depend upon; we crowd other beings out of their niches. Here, on the other hand, is an occasion where our role in biological affairs can be said to be righteously salubrious: we confronted a horrible scourge for centuries; prior generations succeeded in defeating and containing it; and now we are able to ensure that it will never trouble our genus again. In the saga of humans' battles against and cooperation with nature, there are precious few instances in which our ultimate supremacy is so resolutely justified.

A second positive symbol achieved here is the successful marshaling of scientific prowess to thoroughly honorable ends. The overall human record is not unequivocal in this area; there are plenty of instances where our fetish for technology has been exercised in a manner that obscures moral judgments. Is the atom bomb, for example, a net boon or bane for mankind? Are we better off, or worse off, for having accepted the Faustian bargains that produced the internal combustion engine, the television set, and the distillery?

In contrast to those areas of possible moral ambiguity, the antismallpox enterprise offers no such doubts. There is no downside to getting rid of this disease; the symbolism of enlisting technology to our goals is entirely heroic in this case. This story is proof that at least occasionally, human inventiveness and enterprise can mobilize for distinctly positive ends that elevate the entire species and make us proud.

Finally, there is yet another affirmative symbolic act in the form of global political cooperation. The elimination of smallpox could not have been achieved by any one country or one bloc alone. It could not have been accomplished by states operating solely according to the familiar East-West or North-South animus. It was not driven by financial concerns, such as self-interested pursuit of petroleum supplies or the military dominance of outer space. Instead, the struggle against variola has elicited the best in transboundary collaboration; the human spirit has risen to the task, setting aside petty distinctions of race, class, and nationality. People even interrupted wars and other ongoing political struggles in the effort to unite, at least temporarily, against the common problem.

All of these symbols, of course, are already largely in place. The triumph over smallpox has been elevating; eradication of the disease has provided a marvelous case study and, hopefully, a replicable precedent. But the story is not yet quite complete. Only the final eradication of the virus would write the last chapter. Only destruction of those last stocks would make the symbolism perpetual.

REBUTTAL 3: We do not need to destroy variola in order to create another symbol of human triumph over the predatory elements of nature, because we have already accomplished the reality of that triumph via the eradication of smallpox. Now that the disease has been conquered, the point has been made: humans have cooperated in extraordinarily positive ways in our species' triumph over a hostile life-form. People used to die by the millions from smallpox; they no longer do. Nothing we undertake at this point can diminish that accomplishment; nothing more need be done to enhance it. Whether the last few virus samples are incinerated in an autoclave or held indefinitely in a deep freeze, the underlying reality of a smallpox-free world ought to provide all the rhetorical elevation we will ever need.

Moreover, this point about symbolism could be turned on its head. It can be argued that we should hold onto the last variola samples and an array of associated paraphernalia, as "reminders," or symbols, of the tragic past. There is a public education value in the retention—and even in the public display—of this vestige of evil, as providing an occasion to celebrate our shared success, to remember that comparably hazardous pestilence still exists in the world today, and to rededicate ourselves to the same sort of concerted global action that produced this initial victory.

Societies frequently consciously retain visible, compelling artifacts of evil and the struggle against it—people queue up to gaze at Hitler's pajamas, the *Enola Gay*, and Madame Tussaud's waxworks House of Horrors. Perhaps, in that same way, we should preserve a small variola residue to remind everyone of the horrible legacy we have so recently overcome.

ARGUMENT 4: *We no longer need variola for any research or other purposes; we have extracted all the useful lessons that this particular pathogen can teach us.* Earlier proposals to eradicate the virus may have been premature; exhaustive studies of the genetic composition of variola were incomplete, and researchers had not yet gleaned all the information that might be available from it. Within the past couple of years, however, the situation has changed: because of the ongoing research enterprise, now we know (or are on the verge of knowing) all that we will ever need to know about the smallpox virus.

Scientists have completed the genetic map, not just for a single strain of the virus but for ten. These maps would suffice for any plausible scientific needs: for example, the genome roster, rather than the live virus itself, can be the repository used for comparison purposes to reliably identify any similar viruses that might appear in the future. With the maps, novel biological agents can be categorized and cataloged, and future scientific research can continue.

Moreover, we have the ability to retain in useful form the most interesting fragments of the variola DNA, without the attendant risks of intact viruses. The key genes can be parsed, inserted into plasmid loops, replicated, and retained for all manner of study. These controlled conditions can enable researchers to continue their explorations, deciphering any additional messages the viral life processes can convey, without the need to preserve the species as a whole. Thus, even after the eradication of variola, the DNA strands may be able to serve some useful purpose, lending insights into the operation of viruses in general that can aid our struggles against other breeds. But there is no technological need to retain the complete virus for this purpose.

It is worth remembering that today even the intact variola virus, whether encased in CDC freezers, released for tightly controlled microscopic study, or preserved in plasmids, is not the creature in its "natural" state. The only truly natural substrate for variola is the human body; anything else is, by definition, "artificial." Thus, there are practical and theoretical limits to what we can hope to learn from further study of variola. Unless we were (absurdly, unethically) willing to deliberately insert this bug into humans, we could never again fully assess the virus's infective processes, its reproductive prowess, or the finesse with which it identifies and attaches to its specialized cellular targets. Whatever research is still warranted into the functioning of variola, it will of necessity be confined to test tubes; for that type of inquiry, we do not need (and could afford to dispense with the distraction of) the complete virus.

A final observation in this area concerns the importance of continued virology research. One need not be a modern Luddite to oppose additional inquiry into variola. Instead, the argument proceeds from acknowledgment that medical and biological knowledge is far from complete, but it then reaches the conclusion that other diseases, rather than smallpox, merit our concerted action. We already know a great deal about variola; it is time to switch our focus to other, more pressing microscopic enemies. At a time when the viruses associated with AIDS, hantavirus, and Ebola are inflicting death; when influenza is still at large; when legions of other notorious pests deserve our attention, paying attention to yesterday's problems is a misallocation of scarce social resources. Every bit of research devoted to variola, in short, represents an opportunity cost in time, money, and human capital—resources that are not devoted to their highest contemporary demands.

REBUTTAL 4: Two kinds of counterarguments are relevant here. The first challenges the notion that additional variola research has "nothing more to teach us." It contends that no one can truly know what scientific advances—related to smallpox itself, applicable to other areas of virology and immunology, or manifested in completely unforeseen ways—will eventually appear. Because this argument is central to the "affirmative case" that will be constructed in favor of retaining the extant variola stockpiles, it is presented in more detail in chapter 8.

The second counterargument rebuts the notion that usefulness to humans is a necessary criterion for preservation of a species. Even where there is some ambiguity about whether a virus is alive or counts as a recognized species, there is adequate room for challenge to the notion that only by offering some value to human beings does a creature such as variola escape eradication. Just because we are allegedly done with our research into the secrets of variola, does that mean we are free (ethically, legally, etc.) to dispose of it altogether?

Of what use, after all, are other species—the snail darter, the spotted owl? They are not key ingredients in the human food chain; we do not rely upon them as implements of labor. If we make efforts to sustain their existence (efforts that come with substantially greater financial costs than those associated with preserving a few grams of variola), it must be because of some symbolic, ethical, or environmental reasons—and those same rationales would seem to provide an adequate basis for protecting variola. If variola were to surrender its remaining secrets tomorrow through the miracles of microbiological research, does that mean it has forfeited any claim to further existence? Or should we as humans judge things, insentient beings included, along some other moral scale?

ARGUMENT 5:   *Only eradication will permanently eliminate the possibility that smallpox will again be employed as a biological weapons agent.* Smallpox is one of the few potential biological weapons agents that has actually been used for hostile military purposes. The Japanese Special Unit 731 applied it against the Chinese during World War II, and two centuries earlier, British General Amherst may have done likewise against Chief Pontiac. American, Soviet, and other armed forces have explored variola as a possible offensive tool, and the inherent danger cannot be overlooked.

Experts differ as to whether smallpox would be an "optimal" biological agent, or merely a "good" one—the rate of communication, the lethality, and the availability of an effective vaccine may point to other agents with even greater destructive properties. But the world cannot rest easy so long as any potential for deliberate smallpox warfare remains. And today we must add to this volatile mix the power of modern genetic engineering: it may yet prove possible to delicately manipulate the variola genome to steer the bug toward even deadlier, more pernicious directions.

The point is that only by resolutely exterminating all known variola can the world entrench an absolute norm against possession or use, for any reason, at any time. If we were successful in that effort, the message would be communicated that any ownership of this virus, however it came about, was illegitimate. The rules would then mandate immediate destruction of any subsequently discovered samples, whether episodically retrieved from a long-forgotten archive, belatedly discovered by a reformist government, or unearthed by archaeologists. Reaching beyond the question of variola, such actions might prompt a reaffirmation of humankind's shared commitment to avoid all other forms of biological warfare, too, strengthening the Biological Weapons Convention and generating more viable forms of international dispute resolution.

Of course, this sort of leadership by example carries no guarantee. Rogue states or irresponsible substate actors might secretly resist. But global norms can make a difference, even where basic national security interests are at stake. And surely, there is far less chance of inculcating respect for that type of anti-variola standard while some countries (the two military and BW giants) are permitted to retain their stockpiles indefinitely and conduct limitless research upon them.

REBUTTAL 5: Several "arguments in the alternative" are relevant here. First, there may not be any such hidden variola stocks to worry about. None has been discovered in the past two decades; there have been no verifiable hints about secret reserve stashes, whether in rogue states or sloppy laboratories. We cannot be sure, but neither should we allow that small prospect to drive global public policy.

Second, even if the remote possibility of hidden stocks remains, so what? Smallpox might not be a "terrific" biological weapon—for terrorists or regular armies—because of its inherent limitations in persistence, communicability, and so forth, and because of the availability of a global stockpile of efficacious vaccine (which should be preserved and enlarged in any event). Other, better BW agents will continue to be available to the antisocial elements—both the "designer" bugs that could be conceptualized in hostile laboratories and the more commonplace agents that have always survived human efforts at their eradication. The danger of untoward use of biology for warlike purposes will not be abated much by incineration of these few variola stockpiles.

Third, building upon that realpolitik conclusion, there is little logical force to the notion that the possession of a few vials of variola at the CDC and Vector is responsible for perpetuating the specter of biological warfare. A hostile or rogue state or other entity that has husbanded its secret variola reservoir—whether out of fear, suspicion, or the search for one-sided advantage—for all these years is unlikely to be moved to better behavior by our employment of the autoclaves. Whatever we do with these last variola samples, these hypothetical outliers are unlikely to be inspired to come clean.

Finally, if the world continues to be fearful of biological warfare, and dissatisfied about its security against deliberate application of smallpox (or other disease), there is a more direct, efficacious response. Instead of simply destroying this small, militarily insignificant arsenal, we could resolve collectively to strengthen the relevant legal and political standards and institutions. We could upgrade the 1972 Biological Weapons Convention, engraft onto it viable inspection and other verification procedures, and tighten some of its loopholes. We could expand the coverage of customary international law on point, achieving a universal application of the anti-BW norms. We could make continued possession of variola, outside the two licensed facilities, an international crime, with appropriate sanctions on nations or individuals who abuse the prohibitions. We could, in addition, render the illicit possession of smallpox ineffective as a weapon, if our targeted research program ultimately succeeds in its goals of developing improved detectors, vaccines, and antiviral medications to combat the disease. All this could be accomplished without the total eradication of the last few variola samples, and would do much more to ameliorate the perceived dangers.

CONCLUSION

The case for extermination of the last variola stocks suggests that the time has come to draw a curtain across earth's experience with variola. That experience has been profoundly negative: countless millions have lost their lives, their sight, and their families. Even the one small "silver lining," the opportunity for human intellect and enterprise ultimately to triumph over this scourge, remains incomplete. The illness of smallpox has long since been routed, but the causative agent remains in our midst. So long as it persists, the danger of a resurgence is not eradicated, and the costs of safeguarding against such a return are substantial. If ever variola had anything to teach humans, we have now learned those lessons, and we have no further need to tolerate this killer. Therefore, the triumph over smallpox should now be completed through the deliberate extinction of the virus.

тне case against extermination

We turn now to the reverse side of the ledger, presenting the arguments in opposition to the proposition asserted in chapter 7. This chapter should not be interpreted as a plea "in favor of variola," for that creature warrants no advocacy of its own; instead it is simply an assembly of reasons why the proposed elimination, at least at this time, should fail. Again, there are five key arguments, each with its rebuttal.

ARGUMENT 1: *Deliberate extermination of a species is immoral.* The first reason to sustain the variola stockpiles concerns the ethics of preservation. The argument here proceeds not so much from the standpoint of the inherent value of the virus itself, or its key role in nature's grand scheme, but from the degrading effect *on humans* of variola's purposeful extinction. This proposition is simply that it is wrong—in some moral sense that cannot be unpacked much further—to exterminate a species, absent absolutely compelling justification.

Of course, humans have been responsible, directly or indirectly, for the permanent loss of many species. Plants and animals, terrestrial and aquatic, large and small, are disappearing—often without humans' ever being conscious of their presence or their absence. We have not even recognized or begun to catalog many of the species that our civilization routinely tramples. This ongoing streamlining of the planet's biodiversity is at least regrettable; often it may be tragic. And the fact that it is accomplished accidentally, carelessly, or out of monumental ignorance simply compounds the shame.

But with variola, we are approaching something more profound. For the first time, humans will be knowingly and intelligently destroying another species. By acting "with malice aforethought" against one of God's tiniest creatures, we are assuming a role that ill suits our own species. The transition from casual blunderers to self-conscious executioners is a monumental one.

Environmental law—either international accords such as the Biodiversity Convention and CITES, or domestic enactments such as NEPA and the ESA—does not require this degree of self-restraint; those instruments were not crafted with anything like a virus as the objective. Still, the rhetoric of those laws resonates beyond the narrow scope of legally binding mandates, to suggest that in our best moments, when we reflect more deeply on our global long-term interests, we strive to preserve all biodiversity.

This notion of cross-species fair play has its limits, of course. No one would propose that humans attempt to keep hands off nature's realm altogether, as if it could ever be possible for us to avoid all major (and strongly negative) impacts with the environment. Nor could anyone consider it ethical to allow variola to return to its natural state, where it could once again infect and kill humans. Rather, confinement to controlled glass cells seems an appropriate response and ensures that the virus cannot inflict further harm on humans. But going that one monumental step further, deliberately exterminating the race, seems wrong.

The thrust of this argument is not much blunted by the uncertainty over whether a virus deserves to be considered alive, a dispute that itself opens a fascinating window on humans' ability to categorize, organize, and think rigorously about the world around us. But even if variola in some ways more closely resembles a chemical compound such as a hemoglobin molecule, instead of a biological entity, that characterization is hardly binding upon moral theorists. There is something at least lifelike going on with variola, something that is regulated by the Biological Weapons Convention, and the effort to extinguish that trait is morally questionable.

REBUTTAL 1: We have more important things to worry about than the life prospects of this destructive little creature. We have already inflicted enormous violence upon its natural processes, deliberately preventing it from fulfilling its biological objectives (i.e., infecting humans), and confined it to frigid glass—and we have been fully justified in doing so because of the threat it poses to our own species. The primacy of self-preservation amply justifies the further action of destroying the virus altogether, as the only way to ensure that it will pose no renewed threat to humans.

In the case of a virus, in particular, the moral qualms about killing a species are especially misplaced, because this entity is not alive to begin with. Biologically, it is no more than a collection of chemicals, lacking the inherent ability to conduct basic life processes—it has no more right to preservation than does a chunk of concrete or a pool of waste oil. Just as sentimentalists might attempt to preserve an architectural structure simply because it has been around for a long time, as a familiar and salient feature in the local history, some might want to cling to a residue of smallpox. But if the structure is so dilapidated, so contaminated with hazardous materials that it poses a threat to all who enter or merely pass by, and if it cannot be "rescued" or "reformed" in any way, then it should be destroyed as a matter of public safety.

In fact, humans "play God" in this way all the time. We do make social choices that carry profound life-and-death consequences for other beings. That awesome responsibility is inherent in the fact that human beings are, at least for now, the planet's dominant species: what we do about gathering food, improving transportation, multiplying our numbers, and so forth, will inevitably have major repercussions for our fellow planetary inhabitants. We should try to make these fateful decisions intelligently, with respect for the long-term sustainability of the ecosystems we tread upon, but some degree of disruption—and, inevitably, some cases of species extinction—cannot be avoided.

What is different here is the degree of deliberateness applied to the decision to rid the earth of variola. But that self-consciousness is to be celebrated, not condemned. For the first time, humans are attempting to exercise our species' extinction power in a thoughtful, careful, calibrated way, rather than haphazardly. Instead of adopting our usual "reckless" posture that allows other species to slip into extinction with hardly a nod, we are making a positive, debated, and internationally tested choice. We are exercising the best in collective human judgment, wrestling with our responsibilities as stewards of the planet. This careful analysis, global in scale and painstaking in process, is the apotheosis of human intelligent behavior, and a manifestation of respect for the natural world.

ARGUMENT 2: *There may still be lessons to learn from additional variola research—we can never be certain that we have plumbed all the secrets of this virus.* It is arrogance of the highest order to contend that we have already learned everything that can be learned from investigations into variola. Indeed, the essence of true scientific inquiry is the exploration of the unknown—we can never tell what insights may be gained by turning the next corner in research. One is reminded here of the shortsightedness of the nineteenth-century pundits who proposed closing down the U.S. Patent Office, on the grounds that every possible invention had already been developed. Several million patents later, the process is still going strong, and our ability to exploit the mysteries of virology may mushroom in the years to come.

In fact, it is difficult for laypersons to credit at all the notion that science has already extracted all the potential lessons from variola. Surely microbiologists have not learned *everything;* if they had, our species' current struggles against monkey pox, influenza, AIDS, Ebola, and the rest of the viral menagerie would be different. Heterogeneous viruses, of course, have heterogeneous properties, and the transferability of insights from one virus to the next may be limited, but with so many of the fundamental questions about infectivity and human immunity unanswered, it is premature to declare victory.

Additional research conducted solely on fragments of variola DNA might not suffice for these purposes. Even if key segments of DNA are reproduced in plasmids, for example, something interesting might be lost. Having a complete genetic map of the virus might, or might not, tell us everything: if we destroy the original template, we will never know. As one scientist puts it, if you want to learn about the operation of avian flight, it's not sufficient to dissect a bird's wings, its musculature, and its circulatory system in isolation—you have to be able to scrutinize the entire organism in order to understand how the components work together.

This long-term scientific perspective should have a reserved claim on decisions made in the 1990s and early 2000s: if today's scientists, limited by today's research tools and techniques (and, perhaps more significantly, inhibited by contemporary models of virology) cannot ask and answer additional provocative questions about smallpox, perhaps future generations could do better. But they will have an opportunity to stretch their imaginations in this way only if we now act to preserve variola.

It may well be that not much (or any) additional research on variola should be conducted right now. Perhaps the shrewd scientific and medical strategy at this juncture would be to set smallpox aside for a while, to concentrate our attention on, and to deal directly with, the viruses that pose the most pressing dangers for contemporary civilization. But it is prudent at least to return variola to cold storage, preserving the specimens for unknown future contingencies. Why would we throw away—like an unread book—a resource that potentially carries such great scientific value in the future?

REBUTTAL 2: It is difficult to deny that unforeseeable twists in biological researchers' creativity might open new scientific doors in the future. But intelligent policy requires us to calculate the odds. If it is so unlikely that worthwhile information about variola will be revealed, if the probability of fruitful research on this particular creature is so remote, then it may not be worth preserving the opportunity—especially when doing so involves substantial social costs and risks.

We have already conducted a great deal of research on variola—it may be the one virus that has received the largest amount of human attention. We know its biochemical features, its microstructures, and its performance characteristics as well as we know anything in the miniature world. We have drawn successfully upon the lessons we have learned with smallpox to aid us in the battle against other viral pests. But the time has come for researchers to move on: there are other challenges that demand concerted action, and we should approach them directly, focusing our energies on those newly emerging viruses, rather than indirectly, by further working on variola.

ARGUMENT 3: *Respect for global biodiversity, and for the long-term genetic health of the planet, requires us to sustain all manner of creatures, even those with obscure and hostile shreds of DNA.* Humans are only now beginning to realize the importance of the vast biodiversity for a robust, healthy planet. For too long, we have largely taken it for granted, but at last we are awakening to the genetic treasures of proliferating species. Much of the attention to date has focused on the ongoing destruction of the equatorial rain forest, where modern "progress" threatens us all, as high numbers of distinct breeds of flora and fauna are eradicated forever. Much the same appreciation should now apply to the microscopic world, where an even greater array of nucleic acid variability may be found.

Some of these ongoing biodiversity losses may jeopardize humans directly. That is, we depend on plants and animals for our own sustenance—and the more different kinds of companion creatures that are available, the better our long-term prospects are. We can never tell when a new type of fiber or foodstuff can be developed, and we are especially enthralled by the notion that plants and animals may hold the potential as natural factories for elusive pharmaceuticals. An orchid found only beneath the rain forest canopy may distill into a cure for cancer; the immune system of an aquatic mammal may operate in a fashion that sheds new light on our own. Once these species are gone, the opportunity to derive these unique insights and products is lost too.

Admittedly, variola virus serves as a most unlikely "poster child" for the cause of global biodiversity. But who can say from whence our salvation may come? As unappealing as this virus may inherently be, there have already been illustrations of the adaptation of other viruses to noble, even heroic, ends, such as genetically modifying vaccinia to enlist it as a precise carrier of remedial genes in the struggle against horrible illnesses. If we eliminate variola prematurely, we will never know what additional employment it, too, might be turned to in the future.

REBUTTAL 3:   Once again, we have to calculate the likely outcomes, not solely the imaginable ones. That is, it may be barely conceivable that future genetic manipulations could transform variola into a cancer-eating bug, providing a unique boon to our species. And in the same vein, science fiction writers have conjured up visions of aliens from outer space who invade earth, impervious to all our weapons and overwhelming our defenses, but are defeated at the last moment by a simple virus that the human immune system can combat. That, too, is possible, in some far-fetched sense, but it is hardly a basis for sound public policy.

Our reservations in this area are especially justified since it may be just as likely that these deft human attempts at genetic manipulation will backfire. As we try to reformat a virus, to make it a suitable vector for life-sustaining medicines, how do we know that other, insidious alterations are not occurring in tandem—mutations that could unleash a new, even deadlier disease? A sizable number of people suspect that the AIDS virus might have been a human creation—an attempt at just this sort of biodiversity experiment that went crazily awry. That particular conspiracy theory seems misplaced, but the skepticism underlying it, and the grudging respect for nature's chaotic ability to frustrate manifold human efforts at expert manipulation, may be justified. As long as variola exists on earth, and as long as it is a candidate for research and attempts at genetic manipulation, there is a possibility for those experiments to go wrong, perhaps disastrously so.

ARGUMENT 4: *The WHO cannot, in fact, succeed in eliminating all the variola in the world.* The most blunt-edged criticism of the WHO campaign argues that the abolitionists, for all their heartfelt and high-minded sentiments, cannot succeed in eliminating all traces of smallpox materials from the world. Whatever we may collectively do regarding the two known repositories in Atlanta and Koltsovo, we have to acknowledge that these two are only the *known* variola depots. To pretend that we can accomplish more—that we would truly "rid the world of variola forever"—would be perpetrating a fraud, under at least four scenarios.

First, there could be countries (or groups within a country) that have deliberately retained a secret variola inventory. Whether they have done so for hostile purposes or just to "hedge their bets," the lingering stocks represent profound dangers. The history of the secret, illicit Soviet biological warfare facility at Sverdlovsk—and the subsequent Russian pattern of covert BW work continuing for some years, despite the public opposition of Presidents Gorbachev and Yeltsin—substantiate this possibility. Published accounts—based on rumors or on more well-grounded intelligence reports—frequently point at North Korea, Iraq, and other furtive regimes as possible variola possessors.

Second, there could be laboratories that have accidentally or inadvertently kept their smallpox reserves, hidden in the back of a rarely cleaned-out freezer. The combination of poor laboratory techniques, such as inadequate vial labeling, combined with sloppy recording of experimental programs and freezer contents; normal turnover in staff personnel; and imperfect human memories could mean some residual anomalies in compartments that formerly held variola. After all, when smallpox was commonplace, many labs and other facilities held the virus samples for legitimate purposes.

Third, there could still be some viable smallpox virus "in the wild." For more than twenty years, there have not been any outbreaks of the disease in any of the locations where it was formerly endemic, but at least as a theoretical possibility, some latent danger may remain. Scientists have debated whether viable variola might still reside in the corpses of any prehistoric cave dwellers who contracted the disease, died from it, and were frozen in ice grottoes or in approaching glaciers before the virus could dissipate. Upon warming of the area, could the virus be resuscitated? For the most part, the scientific mainstream seems to discount this danger, but in the absence of experience, perhaps we cannot be certain.

Finally, we may be able to " reinvent" variola in the laboratory, even if all natural specimens are destroyed in the autoclaves. This might be achievable through modern genetic manipulation techniques, augmented by the mappings of the various variola genomes (published on the Internet).

Collectively, these scenarios not only drive the conclusion that the WHO eradication campaign would be quixotic in the extreme; they also suggest that it might prove counterproductive. By an act of "unilateral disarmament," in destroying the only legitimate sources of the virus, the world would dramatically increase the value of any covert, illegitimate stocks, reinforcing the incentives that led to their creation, discovery, and retention. Once the U.S. and Russian inventories were disposed of—and with them, the potential opportunity to develop enhanced antismallpox detection, prevention, and treatment materials—the terrorists, rogue scientists, military leaders, and others might well conclude that their covert stocks had progressed from being merely rare to being unique. The world would tremble at the prospect that those outlaws—and only those outlaws—had access to the infective variola materials.

The conclusion, therefore, should be that since we can never be sure that the "bad guys" would no longer possess viable variola, we should not dispose of the last stocks available to the "good guys." We should, instead, retain the materials, and investigate thoroughly—for as long as it might take—the possibilities for improved prevention and treatment, thereby depriving the hostile elements of any value that they might realize from their continued covert possession.

REBUTTAL 4: There is a logical disconnect between the possibility that covert variola stocks might somehow remain or be re-created and the argument that the WHO inventories must be retained. That is, in the highly unlikely event that a rogue state, a hostile military, or a terrorist had stashed away or acquired a smallpox sample, succeeded in weaponizing it, and deployed it as a weapon, there still would be no particular need for the United States, Russia, and their allies and friends to possess smallpox inventories of their own. Even in that extreme event, our response—both militarily and politically—would draw upon the full array of capacities available to the superpowers. We would have the capability to detect and identify the pathogen, we would undertake to develop and apply appropriate isolation and treatment regimens, and we would seek out and defeat the aggressor. Surely, we would never respond "in kind": even if we continued to possess variola of our own, we would not apply those germs in a military fashion. In short, while the world may still lack the capability to anticipate, deter, and deal with a military or terrorist (especially a bioterrorist) threat, continued retention or destruction of the CDC and Vector stocks would be essentially irrelevant to the enterprise.

Moreover, it is appropriate to express considerable skepticism about the notion that further research into variola will yield advances of military relevance. First, science offers no guarantees: no matter how much time, money, energy, and scientific expertise, and how many BL-4 facilities we devote to the problem, we may not succeed in inventing improved vaccines, antivirals, or other materials of practical use against the rogue biological warfare threat. We have leads, hunches, and hypotheses, to be sure, but all these may fizzle—or at least they may prove to be so specific or narrow that a determined aggressor or bioterrorist could continue to leapfrog ahead of us in the molecular offense versus defense arms race.

Second, it is not certain that any sustained variola research program would be continued for the indefinite period of time (and funding) that may be required. Only five years ago (the last time that the variola stocks appeared to be irrevocably positioned on the WHO chopping block), the U.S. military had outlined a conscientious smallpox research plan, driven by the same sorts of fears and expectations that operate today—and that plan quickly slipped beneath the wave of competing budgetary and operational objectives. In 2001 to 2002, the promised research program has at least started in a more concrete and dedicated fashion, but who can say that today's determination will not wane as tomorrow's competing priorities emerge?

ARGUMENT 5: *Before undertaking the deliberate extinction of variola, we should pause to develop sound precedential standards and principles that will be applicable the next time this type of situation arises.* We need to be mindful that in this case, we are not only deciding the permanent fate of the variola virus: we are also setting a precedent that could be followed the next time a species approaches deliberate extinction.

And there will be additional cases. We cannot predict with confidence just which virus, bacteria, or other pest will next stand in the executioner's line, nor can we be certain when that fateful decision will have to be made. But there are other candidates, not that far away. Poliomyelitis—the dreaded scourge of childhood in the late 1940s and early 1950s—for example, has now essentially disappeared from the Western Hemisphere, and efforts to eradicate it globally are proceeding apace. That virus is just as hated as smallpox and possesses just as few redeeming qualities. Likewise, the pathogens causing leprosy, measles, guinea worm fever, and maybe tuberculosis could be next.

Human beings are therefore consigned to being "repeat players" in the business of deliberate extinction. We will, one way or the other, decide the fates of additional miniature creatures in the decades to come: some viruses, some other germs that fulfill more traditional biological criteria for "living" beings. Our experience with variola is far from an isolated instance.

How should we, as a species, think about the preservation or destruction of other species? What rules/procedures should we apply? What standards decide who shall live and who shall perish? Is this properly a decision of the World Health Organization and its associated scientific and medical experts, or should other bodies and individuals play a role? How much should we be moved by the potential ongoing "utility" (or lack thereof) of a particular species? Does it matter whether the creature is a potential (or actual) biological warfare agent? Do we differentiate between those pathogens that cause deadly diseases (e.g., the AIDS virus) and those that are more often nonfatal?

Are we making an impetuous decision, reached in elation's heat upon the triumph over a dreaded disease? Would we act differently, if we were to pause for more sober reflection upon the enduring standards, both substantive and procedural, that we would seek to employ prospectively? This decision, in the case of variola, is irrevocable, as are its implications for the human future. Social decision making is always a challenge; trying to act on the basis of urgency, without a carefully derived protocol that we would stand by in future cases, is not the wise way to proceed.

REBUTTAL 5: This is hardly a hasty act. The WHO has been pondering the final eradication of smallpox for two decades. The decision to destroy the virus, initially made in 1986, has been delayed, rethought, and reaffirmed on multiple occasions. Every opportunity for second thoughts and changed attitudes has been allowed. If anything, the international mechanism has hesitated excruciatingly while considering all the arguments and counterarguments. It is now clear that most of the world would stand behind an extermination decision, and we can embrace it as a model of meticulously careful, global consensus-building. If this pattern is repeated in the future, with the polio virus or any other disease-causing microbe, we will know that we have done our best to think through all the alternatives and reach the best outcome.

Moreover, the precedential impact of the variola decision should not be overstated. There are not, after all, so many cases that might come up—at least not in the immediate future. And each one of them will be unique, offering its own array of fateful options and competing concerns. Some viruses may merit additional research; some might offer real promise for pharmaceutical applications. In some cases, the security concerns will be less threatening; in others, the fears of a possible escape could be even greater. We do not so much need general principles and standards to deal with these unique cases when they arise; instead, we need a commitment—readily evidenced in the case of smallpox—to think through the issues carefully, to study all the variables, and to ponder our options before we act.

We should not, after all, romanticize this problem. Variola is a nonliving creature that has killed people for centuries; if we can protect ourselves from it, that is morally justified and perhaps morally required. Other microbes may present different problems and opportunities in the future, but variola is the easiest case among them.

CONCLUSION

The case against extermination suggests that we can do better than eradicate variola—better for ourselves and for our posterity. It is an affirmation of our humanness to find alternatives other than extinction, even for this confirmed enemy of our species. Both a utilitarian calculus (the possibility that future uses may yet be found for the virus, and the possibility that further research upon it may teach us lessons that we can apply in our struggles against other infections) and a moral reasoning (the notion that people have an obligation to preserve the biological diversity of the planet, including when noxious pathogens are concerned) should lead us in this direction. This is not a plea for mercy for variola—it should still be housed only in the most controlled, secure laboratories, and any research on it must be carefully safeguarded. But there is no need to destroy the species; we should, instead, hold on to it "just in case."

CHAPTER 9

CONCLUSIONS AND RECOMMENDATIONS

DEALING WITH DANGER

Uncertainty and risk are inherent, and inherently troublesome, in human life. Too often, we fail to appreciate the full range of options available to us, we err in our calculations of the probabilities of outcomes, and we misapprehend the costs and benefits of each course.

Problems such as smallpox are especially frustrating in this regard, as it proves ineffably strenuous to stretch our minds, and our social institutions, around the complexity of the issue. Perhaps one way to approach smallpox, therefore, taking at least one step toward a beginning of knowledge, is to catalog frankly some of the impediments to rational social choice here. If we are explicit about the difficulties in deciding intelligently what to do about variola extermination, perhaps that confession itself can indicate a path.

First, the issue is difficult because of its novelty. We have no precedents of deliberate extinction, no models to help shape our thinking, and no relevant experience to serve as a "reality check" on our instincts. Second, the problem is complex, drawing upon the insights, doctrines, and methodologies of distinct disciplines—the various dimensions surveyed in this book. The third consideration is urgency: there is a timetable, albeit a slippery one, imposed by the

World Health Organization, requiring action (or further delay) if not in 2002, then at intervals thereafter.

Fourth, that action would be final: once the Georgia and Novosibirsk samples are sent to the autoclave, there is no turning back. Fifth, the stakes are high: these days, nothing excites the passions—legitimately—more than the specter of biological warfare and terrorism. Sixth, the experts disagree: the scientific literature abounds with their sharply worded disputes about the value of future research on the samples, the trustworthiness of the various institutional players, and the morality of abolition. If the experts are so divided, within the core areas of their scientific expertise, how can the rest of us contribute to the discussion?

Most of all, the problem is confounded by the incommensurability of the various risks. How are we to compare such different types of hazards and opportunities; how are we to think coherently about riddles that require us to trade off such distinct values, each one of which is sufficiently complicated and unknown even on its own "home turf"?

Here, we have somehow to weigh in the balance:

the risk that as long as the smallpox virus is retained, it might somehow escape, by accident or evil design, from the Russian and American deep freezes and spread devastating disease;

the opportunity to glean novel insights into viral operations and human responses, perhaps leading to improvements in areas from influenza vaccination to suppression of the body's rejection of organ transplants;

the scenarios of deliberate biological warfare and bioterrorism emanating from some country's hidden stockpiles, especially if aided by a chimera virus incorporating a genetically enhanced variant of variola;

the moral questions centered on playing God or Frankenstein as we manipulate the genomes of various creatures, possibly creating new forms of life and extinguishing old ones;

the politics of international relations within the respected but still troubled halls of the World Health Organization, where the familiar tensions between East and West, and between North and South, are played out against the backdrop of global medical campaigns;

the necessity of safeguarding former Soviet biological weapons facilities, materials, and expertise, to convert them to peaceful uses and interdict an incipient brain drain of biological weaponeers onto the international black market;

the apprehension that frozen variola remnants, somehow rescued from ice age cadavers, might be revivified, by happenstance or concerted effort; and

the possibility that the unique coding of variola's DNA might hold, for future generations of researchers, as well as for nature itself, a biodiversity value that we cannot imagine today.

In general, human beings seem not very skilled at thinking about such unwieldy arrays of risk, particularly when so many of the elements fit into the category of low probability of occurrence but high impact if they do occur. Especially when the time horizon is so extended, when any payoff would be realized long after completion of the next election cycle, one cannot expect the Congress or the executive branch to eagerly fund and carefully supervise work on the remote contingencies.

Even the precautionary principle, which is becoming a touchstone in certain areas of environmental law, seems incomplete here, where it is debatable which course of action would be truly safer. Do we demonstrate regard for the interests of ourselves and our posterity by destroying the variola samples immediately, to ensure that future generations will never be exposed to smallpox? Or do we instead preserve the residues, with appropriate safeguards, to ensure that our successors will have access to this unique viral entity for research and exploitation purposes that are beyond contemporary ken?

Reliance upon the usual array of democratic procedures also seems misplaced here. For some reason, this doesn't quite seem the sort of question best resolved through ordinary voting, with the peoples of the world represented according to a one country, one vote system in the World Health Assembly. But it also doesn't seem to be a matter in which the accident of historical possession of the last two stockpiles should confer upon the United States and Russia sole de facto authority to decide an issue of such great moment for all. The other countries of the world, who each have a stake in the outcome and who each played a tragic/heroic role in battling the disease, may well resent the unilateral U.S. approach to this global issue.

DEALING WITH POLITICS

The politics of the smallpox question are similarly convoluted. Each bloc, each country, each decision maker is pulled in different directions. At the macrolevel, developing countries (including those who suffered the most and the longest from smallpox) may wonder why the global variola inventories (some of which they themselves had sent to Atlanta or Moscow) should remain under the control of the two nations that dominated the unlamented cold war era. Likewise each country must come to appreciate the multidimensional character of the dilemma; it is no accident that the repeated pattern reveals the respective ministries of defense inclined to want to retain the virus repositories while the ministries of health favor abolition.

If we think of this issue as being fundamentally a problem of public health, then the most appealing avenue might be to rid ourselves forever of a dangerous pathogen, especially one against which our natural and institutional defenses have lapsed. But if we conceptualize this issue with national security as the frame of reference, then the concept of unilateral disarmament seems counterintuitive, especially in face of the mounting apprehensions about biological terrorism and rogue states. From other initial perspectives, those who approach the issue from a starting point grounded in environmentalism's respect for biodiversity, or from an ethical or religious orientation, might shy away from exercising the power to destroy the last vestiges of a unique creature that has somehow survived millennia. And a microbiologist's predilection would routinely be to retain such a fascinating creature for further, as yet undefined, study.

There is at least one way in which the variola question is less complicated than it might otherwise be: there is not a lot of money at stake. To be sure, there is some cash on the table: some researchers will get projects funded or not, some vaccine procurement programs will be supported more than others, and the levels of assistance that America provides to the Vector laboratory in Koltsovo might wax or wane. But that is "small potatoes" compared to what the economic costs can be when endangered species are to be protected, when genetic engineering technology is questioned, or when defense industries are preserved. This is not an issue that displaces shopping centers and highways, that implicates oil reserves, or that promises one country or one organization special access to unique secrets of outer space or the deep sea.

The September 11, 2001, terrorist attacks and the subsequent flurry of mailed anthrax spores reveal yet another insidious aspect of the current controversy. Like the anthrax bacillus, variola is an exquisitely dangerous bioterrorism agent: it is silent, invisible, and deadly. But smallpox goes beyond anthrax, in being communicable from person to person. That reality compounds the dangers and the social vulnerability: once a terrorist or rogue nation has successfully infiltrated variola virus into a community, the virus can proliferate through the timeless biological mechanisms of infection, reproduction, and dissemination. The threat, at that point, comes not from a suspicious package or the mail system but from other human beings. Any person—not just a mysterious militant or domestic sociopath but even your family, friends, coworkers—can become an unwitting "ally" of the terrorists, conveying the virus to new targets and intensifying the potential for public panic, rage, and fear.

The smallpox story, viewed in historic terms, is a unique saga of human triumph: in those few decades of the twentieth century, humans temporarily set aside some of their worst political differences, and some of their ongoing wars, to unite behind a global vaccination campaign. The collaboration was an immense success, when measured in monetary terms, in the number of lives saved, and in the level of international cooperation achieved. If the human species can accomplish that level of greatness in moments of high peril, perhaps some of that unity can be sustained as we confront the lingering question of what to do with the variola residuals.

RECOMMENDATIONS

In closing, I offer the following recommendations, as simply one effort to reconcile the many dimensions of the variola question.

1. Retain the current variola stocks

I would keep the virus, for two reasons. First, I would hold onto this unique resource "just in case." I don't have a compelling answer to the logical follow-up question "In case of what?" But I do retain the naive confidence that future generations will conjure uses for even noxious substances that we devalue today. The medical models available to us now are not timeless; perhaps tomorrow's researchers will be able to ask better questions, apply improved technology, and obtain more interesting results than our current puny efforts have. They may be able to recycle the variola genome, bending it to more productive and instructive applications that would be foreclosed forever if we pull the plug on the virus today.

In starting with that "utilitarian" viewpoint, however, I am not motivated solely by the future value to humans of the viral entity. I would also prefer to keep the virus because it seems like the right thing to do. Deliberate extermination, even of a competing species, seems arrogant; it is not the sort of move that human beings should be comfortable making. Especially where the inherent dangers of preservation can be managed with appropriate security and safety protocols, it is a cost our species should bear. I do not feel any sympathy for the execrable virus, I am not, at the bottom line, moved to protect its claimed right to existence. But something—if not mercy, then perhaps respect for another life-form—motivates me to conclude that where coexistence is possible (with the predator entombed in frozen glass), it is morally preferable. The rhetoric and spirit (if not the precise coverage and operational terms) of domestic and international environmental law enactments such as the Biodiversity Convention and the Endangered Species Act have it right—species are per se worth preserving.

Notably, I would not be motivated to maintain the stocks simply because of the possibility that someone else (North Korea, Iraq, China, etc.) may also have secret supplies. While that danger does call for prompt additional research on improved mechanisms for detection, protection, and treatment, our shields against rogues and terrorists in the long term must depend fundamentally on other strengths. We have to rely upon intelligence capabilities, diplomacy, military strength, deterrence, and the like—certainly not on the possibility of retaliation in kind. This is one of the few situations where the concept of unilateral self-restraint makes sense; we do not need our own variola stocks in order to identify any future viruses or to figure out how to deal with the evildoers. The threat of bioterrorism, in short, should energize our research, intelligence, defense, and political establishments but should not by itself compel us to hold onto variola forever.

2. Retain the stocks indefinitely, without a fixed timetable

We are currently in something of a use it or lose it mentality regarding variola. That is, unless the United States and Russia proceed diligently forward with their announced research programs, pursuing short-term goals of improved vaccines, treatments, and detectors, there is every indication that pressures will mount within the WHO system to advance toward eradication. And that research does make sense; those are admirable, important goals, and if (by some miracle) the investigators can accomplish them in the near term, so much the better.

But science typically does not proceed strictly according to the programmers' announced timetables; it make take longer—perhaps much longer—to achieve the kinds of breakthroughs that would enhance our security against the terrorist, rogue, or other biological warfare threats. Especially now that the United States has profoundly upped the ante regarding the goals of the research program—we now seek not one but two antivirals, as well as a new vaccine and a fistful of additional goals—any projection of a laboratory timetable is conjectural at best. What we need is not a short duration "crash" program, butting up against an artificial deadline, but a more studied, systematic approach, defining the research opportunities that present themselves and pursuing them in a rigorous, prudent fashion, detached from the political pressures in Geneva.

It may take years to reveal the secrets that variola now conceals. And it may be that some of the most interesting and productive research cannot be initiated until science, over time, develops the appropriate tools, concepts, and techniques. Sometimes, the best use of a resource, the most cleverly designed research protocol, is simply to do nothing—to husband the stockpile, ensuring that it will remain viable until our successors are better able to exploit it for the future.

For that reason, I would urge the WHO not to invoke additional artificial deadlines for variola destruction. We may need to retain the virus indefinitely, perhaps forever—no one can now promise when we will truly be finished decoding all its potential secrets. Instead of a "rush to failure," we should undertake a diligent research program now but also understand that the payoff may be long delayed. A wise course would be to decide in favor of indefinite retention, rather than setting a new "due date" for destruction, but mandate periodic review of that choice at, say, ten-year intervals. These reappraisals could decide whether sufficient new developments (political, technical, medical, etc.) warrant a reversal of the decision about variola's fate.

3. Proceed with a judicious research program

Some of the current research does seem worthwhile and should be continued. The fears about incipient bioterrorism are real; the consequences, should some rogue regimes or individuals acquire variola, could be catastrophic. Remarkably, medicine does offer the prospect, through adequate diagnostic, prophylactic, and treatment routines, of creating a "cure" to the threat of biological warfare—a lofty goal that is unimaginable in the case of nuclear or conventional attack.

It has been so difficult to gear up the domestic and international medical/biological apparatus to initiate this smallpox research—acquiring the funds, personnel, and BL-4 laboratory time for the purpose—that we should take advantage of the opportunity. Even if it seems unrealistic to expect the program to achieve its goals within the short time allocated, the good start already made should not be squandered, and the investigations should proceed forward at a serious, diligent pace.

The objectives of the research program remain essentially what they have been for over a decade: to develop improved detection and diagnostic equipment and procedures; to create a safer, equally effective vaccine; and to find or invent a robust antiviral agent. In the first instance, variola is the immediate target of these inquiries, but both a broader appreciation for the needs of national security and public health, as well as a sense of where the commercial market lies, should encourage efforts that may carry applications for other viruses. This will probably and indefinitely remain in large part a federal government effort, but the private sector should also be encouraged to seek remunerative opportunities.

The U.S. Food and Drug Administration is a key player because the usual routine for the development of a new pharmaceutical—including extensive human trials—will not be possible with a disease like smallpox. Accordingly, greater reliance than usual will have to be vested in indirect experiments—proceedings in vitro, or with animal disease models that only approximate smallpox. The FDA (and its counterparts in other countries) will have to walk a narrower tightrope than usual, responding to the emergent needs by facilitating swift evaluation of new candidate pharmaceuticals while still preserving a margin for the safety and efficacy of anything marketed to combat smallpox.

But the bar for research should not be set impossibly high. For example, the goal of developing two antiviral medications that would attack variola through biologically independent mechanisms is probably an example of "overkill." As important as antivirals are, they would likely play only a limited role in combating a smallpox outbreak. Because the existing vaccine is effective even if given shortly after exposure, and because the primary strategy for confronting an outbreak would be the proven surveillance/containment strategy—combating the disease by prompt identification and isolation of each case, accompanied by swift and comprehensive vaccination of all people in the victim's immediate circle—antivirals would be useful for only a small number of initial exposures. Postexposure protection is, therefore, worth pursuing, but not at all costs.

In the same vein, we should be careful not to "hype" the threat. Although we need to respond to the specter of biological warfare and terrorism, we are not defenseless even today. Without the improved antivariola vaccines, treatments, and detectors, we still have a vast array of political, military, and medical tools at our disposal, and any potential aggressor would likely be deterred by the formidable challenges. By the same token, if our antismallpox inquiries were somehow to yield overnight success, that would hardly be the end of the BW threat. Even if we could permanently remove smallpox from the roster of potential biological agents of interest to renegades, there would still be many other viral, bacterial, and other pathogens to fill our nightmares and empty our defense budgets.

4. Continue to involve the experts, but be careful about what we ask them

The smallpox controversy presents a case study of successful use of expert committees. At the international level, decades of standing, special, and ad hoc committees have rendered extraordinary service to the World Health Organization and the general public. They have scrutinized the dangers of continued retention, the opportunities for further research, and the modalities for possible exploitation of the virus. On the national level, the National Academy of

Science's Institute of Medicine has provided highly respected, timely, nonideological guidance for decision making.

Some of those committees, however, appear to have been narrowly constructed. The weighty WHO Ad Hoc Committee on Orthopoxvirus Infections contained only ten members, including three Americans, two Russians, and two Britons. Most of them have been members of the committee for a long time, with no input of "fresh blood." While there is no need—in fact, it would be a grievous mistake—to insist upon term limits or rigid geographical distribution for expert committees of this sort, it is important to avoid perpetuation of any tightly networked "old boys' club."

Moreover, the mandates for these groups should continue the practice of specifying exactly what queries to pose to the groups. The 1999 IOM committee, for example, was explicitly not asked to opine on the ultimate question about what to do with the variola stocks; it was asked, instead, to provide input regarding possible future research applications. Likewise, WHO has (at least most of the time) given its subsidiary bodies specific charges—to monitor the research, to inspect facility safety and security, and so on—appropriately reserving for the senior policy-level bodies (the executive board and the assembly) the power to reach the ultimate decisions. This practice should be continued; it suitably draws upon experts for their unique input, while not excessively delegating political power to them.

In the same vein, we should appreciate that the decision about the variola stocks is not essentially—or not exclusively—a health issue. The WHO is an appropriate body to play the leading role in this global decision making, and it must remain at the epicenter of the controversy, but other institutions should participate too. This is partially a security issue, partially an environmental issue, partially a legal issue, and partially a moral issue, so other affiliates of the United Nations should be pressed into service, and the corresponding national ministries inside many individual countries should be engaged. The rest of the international stakeholding constituencies cannot wash their hands of an aliquot share of responsibility for this policy choice.

Furthermore, something akin to the environmental impact statement process might be useful. There is no need for hundreds of additional pages of scientific analysis of the ecological impacts of variola extermination, since by now, those are largely either: (a) obvious (in that the intention is to eradicate the entire species) or (b) unknowable (in that we can only speculate about what future scientific research might unlock). But the effort, required by NEPA in so many other situations, to engage multiple disciplines would be a welcome expansion of the sole concentration of the issue in the hands of microbiologists and virologists. More of the general public's attention for this controversy would also be welcome; while there is a great deal to be said for expertise in resolving this issue, ultimately it is a social or cultural choice too, and the full body politic ought to participate.

5. Restrict, monitor, and publicize the variola research and facilities

The WHO has not authorized open-ended research on variola; only particular types of inquiries, aimed at particular types of objectives, have been approved. Restrictions of this sort—defining who can undertake what programs, where, and with what protections—are essential, to avoid both the danger of misuse and the equally problematic appearance of misuse. The program should be carefully monitored by authoritative inspectors, and the results should be published and widely disseminated, for whatever peaceful applications countries may seek to employ. Researchers from any country ought to be able to participate in the investigations, sharing the opportunities to learn and to contribute to the learning of others. And, of course, the facilities where the research is occurring—at the CDC, the Vector lab, or elsewhere—must comply with the highest standards of safety and security, consistent with the attendant dangers.

International transparency in the research will help ensure that the United States and Russia are not (and are not perceived, thought, or feared to be) exploiting a unique global resource for special national purposes or seeking a one-sided military advantage in biological warfare or defenses. In the same vein, the WHO and its leading participants should commit now to some fair system for global sharing of the benefits to be derived from this licensed research. We should not allow market forces alone to determine who has access to smallpox vaccine during a crisis; the global permission for retention and experimentation upon the virus samples should not be distorted into a process that differentially protects the United States, Russia, and Europe while once again exposing the developing countries, who have always suffered the most from the disease.

There is, of course, risk in this openness. Malevolent actors might be able to gather militarily useful information and divert it to terrorist or other hostile purposes. If our inquiries produce new vaccines, perhaps they will also suggest ways to circumvent those vaccines; if we generate improved detectors and antiviral medications, perhaps the rogues can also derive countermeasures that will assist an act of aggression. No medical or biological information is so "pure" that it cannot be diverted to harmful ends.

This is the occasion to think anew about our publication strategy. It could be seen as shortsighted, even suicidal, to assist terrorists by describing in detail, and publishing on the Internet, the instructions on how they could best surmount the practical and technical difficulties that have traditionally impeded biological warfare. Yet at the same time, there is no salvation in censorship and compartmentalization: the free flow of information is essential to our prosperity, our inventiveness, and perhaps our survival. We may simply have to hope that the benevolent side of the research can progress at least as fast as the "leakage" of the information to potentially evil applications, and we should attempt to wield our other security assets to help make it so.

6. Maintain and build up inventories of antismallpox materials and expertise

Until the research program achieves its crowning successes, we will have to continue to deal with the world of potential biological warfare as it now is, and prudence dictates that we maintain—or, in some cases, create or enhance—suitable stockpiles of equipment, materials, and know-how that would be essential in responding to a smallpox outbreak today.

In the first instance, this means returning to some of the original 1980 recommendations of the WHO Global Commission for the Certification of Smallpox Eradication, to preserve an adequate inventory of viable vaccine. This commitment, originally ensuring at least 200 million doses worldwide, has unwisely been allowed to atrophy, and no one is sure exactly how many doses of vaccine remain and how potent they still are. The U.S. Departments of Health and Human Services and of Defense stepped up to this danger in the late 1990s, contracting for production of 40 million new doses over sixteen years. After September 11, 2001, the order was increased to 50 million doses, with delivery expedited to 2002. These were important steps in the right direction, initiatives that other countries and the WHO should emulate.

Quantities of suitable delivery systems, either jet injectors or bifurcated needles, should also be stockpiled, because in an emergency there would not be sufficient time to begin new production. For the same reason, physicians or other health workers should be trained now to use that specialized equipment, so they will not have to receive the introductory orientation during a time of crisis. Vaccinia immune globulin (VIG), necessary to treat the rare cases of adverse reaction to the vaccine, should also be generated and preserved in quantity, as the supply of this chemical is now so low that vaccination programs could not be safely reinitiated. And throughout the process, the responsible organizations should take greater care in the stewardship of the stocks, monitoring their condition, testing their potency, and ensuring reliable constancy in conditions such as varying temperature and humidity. Again, following the original WHO recommendations, the inventory (and suitable seed stocks, enabling manufacture of more vaccine) ought to be distributed to at least two dispersed facilities, to guard against catastrophic failure in one.

For similar reasons, the security of the existing variola stockpiles in Atlanta and Koltsovo should be reassessed, including consideration of their susceptibility to such dangerous scenarios as suicidal aircraft hijackings. And it makes sense to tighten down on "gray market" access to dangerous pathogens: the regulations on culture collections and other supply houses should do more to ensure that purchasers of dual capability biological materials will not divert them to antisocial purposes. This objective will require international cooperation of the highest order, to license each country's vendors—there are hundreds of potential sources for these substances worldwide—to inspect their facilities, monitor their shipping protocols, and ensure that they do business only with legitimate purchasers.

But recent events have also demonstrated that it is possible to overreact: no idea is so good, no safety precaution is so sound, that it cannot be carried too far. The Bush administration's October 2001 proposal for a "crash" program to amass 300 million doses of smallpox vaccine—enough to treat every American—within a year provides a vivid illustration of such well-meaning but excessive zeal.

We do not need 300 million doses of vaccinia. We would never administer that many injections, given the number of people with serious contraindications. Too many illnesses and hundreds of deaths would result from returning to the comprehensive approach that public health officials prudently abandoned twenty-five years ago. Moreover, even in the eventuality of smallpox outbreaks, the surveillance/containment strategy was proven superior during the WHO global smallpox eradication campaign. As mentioned earlier, vaccination, even within a few days after exposure, provides protection, and that, rather than indiscriminate treatment of everyone, would be the suitable approach.

In sum, augmented quantities of an improved vaccine should be generated but administered only to at-risk populations—researchers, maybe some primary health care workers, perhaps some military special forces. But the general public in the United States or elsewhere should not now be vaccinated, either on a mandatory or voluntary basis.

Recent simulation exercises such as 2001's Dark Winter have succeeded in portraying more vividly our potential vulnerability to a smallpox terrorist incident, and the expert groups have boosted their estimates of the appropriate size of a safe national vaccine inventory from 40 million doses to perhaps 100 to 135 million. The rest of the world, too, should augment its vaccine pool—although, again, manufacturing one dose for every person would be a terribly wasteful appropriation of scarce funds that could more profitably be devoted to other public health applications.

There is a "security blanket" effect in being able to advise the public that 100 percent vaccine coverage is available: people may be less apprehensive about the prospect of a smallpox attack, and in an era of bioterrorism worries, reassurance is valuable. (The best outcome, of course, would be the development of a new kind of vaccine to be safer and carry fewer adverse side effects—that remains a primary goal on the international research agenda.) But in the short term, it would be a more effective strategy, doing more to achieve the reality of safety (rather than simply the image of protection) to devote the time, attention, and funds to more genuine public health needs, instead of accumulating a redundant, overly endowed vaccinia stockpile.

Just as important is streamlining the delivery system, to ensure that adequate quantities of high-quality vaccine and trained personnel could be dispatched to any locale anywhere around the world on short notice. Instrumental to that objective, the global procedures for identifying and reporting suspicious outbreaks of poxlike illnesses must be maintained and upgraded; where the absence of recent emergencies has allowed these capacities to atrophy, they should now be reinforced. The ongoing experiments with improvements in the WHO's International Health Regulations should be finalized promptly; reinvigorating the procedures for communicating about dangerous illnesses (and about symptoms that could be indicative of such communicable diseases) should be a top priority.

7. Address the burgeoning bioterrorism threat directly

Much has been written lately about the imperative for responding to the radically altered post-cold-war international security environment, in which the threat of terrorism—especially as exemplified by a new breed of exceptionally ambitious, disciplined, and powerful nonstate actors, perhaps armed with biological weapons—seems to be a prominent new feature. In the area of smallpox, in particular, our guard needs to be raised. If there are variola inventories hidden outside the Atlanta and Koltsovo WHO facilities, we need to know about them—an extraordinarily ambitious tasking for our intelligence community. We must pursue improved threat assessment, to discern in advance what sorts of attacks the malefactors may be planning—this, too, requires augmented "human intelligence" assets (i.e., spies) in a field where that sort of inside source has been very difficult to recruit and sustain.

The nature of "asymmetrical warfare" is that the shrewd opponent will not strike us where we are strong but where our vulnerabilities can be exploited, which may mean that the homeland civilian economy and social institutions are jeopardized as never before. We must gear up for possible variants in national security threats and must organize our capabilities to confront the new paradigms. Better cooperation among federal agencies (State, Defense, Federal Emergency Management Agency, Homeland Security, etc.) and between local, state, and federal responders will be essential to this task. Improved ability to detect and identify BW droplets promptly—in a cloud, on a mailed parcel, at a restaurant salad bar, or in any other guise—will be critical. Once the pathogen is detected, improved decontamination agents, procedures, and equipment will be needed. To some extent, these materials and routines may have to be germ specific, but to some extent the antivariola precautions can serve to protect the community from diverse other BW threats, as well.

8. Think of these stocks (and future cases of similar defeated pathogens) as global, not national, resources

For historical reasons, the effort to concentrate the world's variola inventories into a small number of WHO collaborating centers eventually reduced the known stocks to just the superpowers' two. And for equally understandable reasons, the lion's share of responsibility for determining the fate of those last test tubes has fallen to Washington and Moscow. That will likely continue to be a reality for variola, but it need not be the invariant model for dealing with residual stocks of polio virus or other pathogens the world is eventually able to extirpate from the human environment.

In fact, the next time the world approaches the brink of species eradication—which could be the situation for polio within the next few years—a different, more inclusive model ought to be followed. The materials should not necessarily be held only by the two military giants; an international repository, located in a neutral country, might be more suitable. Also, if the pathogen is to be retained for experimental purposes, perhaps multinational facilities would be the appropriate locations for the research, rather than places within the sole jurisdiction of any one country.

We have few good models of this type of international scientific cooperation, in the field of arms control or elsewhere. Implicit in them is some sort of partial surrender of state sovereignty, to allow authoritative decisions to be made by international institutions outside any one state's control. It may still not be easy to create and preserve such transcendent entities, but it is worth the effort here.

Obviously, the power, technological sophistication, and resources of the United States and Russia would continue to make them the leading—probably the essential—players in the unfolding global drama, but in the future it would be better to conceptualize this sort of issue from the start as an occasion for nondiscriminatory global, rather than unilateral national, action. The United States has too often demonstrated a go-it-alone philosophy, making a solo national decision—most vividly, the November 2001 declaration that America will not destroy the variola stocks held at the CDC—and trying, after the fact, to "sell" the result to the rest of the world. That is a formula for inspiring resentment by other countries, other stakeholders in the matter, and it is both unnecessary and unwise as a vehicle for decision making.

9. Enhance the concept that unauthorized possession and use of variola are criminal

Fundamental to the abolitionists' argument is the notion that ostentatious destruction of the two known variola stocks would constitute the clearest public statement that possession—and, a fortiori, hostile use—of these biological materials would be unacceptable. The world would formally and vividly declare that smallpox is totally "out of bounds," and that any continued retention, under any guise whatsoever, is contrary to the most deeply held community values.

I believe, however, that the world can make virtually the same statement, with virtually the same emphasis and power, while retaining the two repositories under strict, internationally monitored conditions. We could employ existing or new legal tools to propound the antivariola and anti-BW messages with great vigor and determination.

We should, for example, enhance the verification and inspection capabilities of the 1972 Biological Weapons Convention and amend it to specify that any possession of this pathogen, outside WHO auspices, is illegal. In this regard, the U.S. opposition to the draft protocol to the treaty should be rethought, or at least efforts should be redoubled to develop a new mechanism for policing BW-related programs more effectively, without unduly inhibiting commercial and research activity—and perhaps that balance should now be struck somewhat differently from before September 11, 2001.

We should also craft a new treaty to institute domestic or international systems of criminal and civil liability for unauthorized possession or use of biological weapons materials. Likewise, we should entrench within the customary or treaty-based international law of armed conflict an intensified notion that hostile application of variola is a crime against humanity, a crime of universal jurisdiction, validly subject to enforcement action by any country. We should also require all countries to search their laboratory inventories and archives thoroughly and declare authoritatively that they possess no variola residues.

Next, we should reinforce our current self-defense capabilities by strengthening the training of, and providing additional equipment to, the local first responders who would constitute the front lines in any effort to deal with an incident of domestic variola terrorism. Their abilities to identify, isolate, treat, and decontaminate afflicted persons would surely be crucial to any effort to react effectively, swiftly, and safely to the attack. Years without the occasion to diagnose a single case of smallpox have led to a diminished capability in the health care system to recognize variola at work; that deficit should be repaired for both emergency room staff and general practitioners. We should find ways to take advantage of modern capabilities for electronic communications and distance learning to propagate better understanding of microbial threats— Websites and associated training materials can educate professionals swiftly and effectively about the modern iteration of a variola threat.

Advanced technical detectors, to sniff out biological pathogens in the environment (especially in locations of mass assembly, such as airports, subways, sports stadiums, and large office buildings), should be a priority. Mechanisms to link together the various first responders—to upgrade the alert status of the entire nation's public health system—would also be crucial. The training and equipment for all affected groups will have to be enhanced to be attentive to forensic needs: the first responders are not only managing the emergency health needs of the affected persons; they may also be, for better or worse, the initial custodians of a crime scene and must be attentive to the mandate to collect and preserve evidence that could be admissible in a criminal prosecution and persuasive in the court of world public opinion.

Public education plays a role too: the nonexpert public should be better informed about the bioterrorism threat in general and about smallpox in particular. A community more able to recognize and respond intelligently to genuine threats will be less prone to overreaction and panic, achieving an attitude of poise that is itself something of a deterrent to terrorism.

All this could be accomplished even if the two stockpiles were retained, and even if WHO-authorized research were allowed to continue indefinitely. That approach does lack something of the comprehensiveness, the absolutism that complete extermination of variola would allow, and nothing expresses our moral position as emphatically as extinction. But much, if not most, criminal law is inherently somewhat ambivalent in this same way: we outlaw speeding, except for ambulances in emergency; we prohibit homicides in general, but allow capital punishment and authorized military actions; we have a widely held norm against private possession of superdangerous devices such as nuclear weapons, but we nonetheless allow the U.S. government and a few others to continue to deploy them. Perhaps those partial prohibitions and semipermeable mandates lack the resounding clarity of "no possession by anyone at any time for any purpose," but that seems to be a tolerable fact of complex modern life.

10. Continue research into related fields and attempt to develop and exploit the synergies

Inquiries into variola, as important as they may be, should not be conducted in isolation. Researchers currently exploring other pox diseases—from monkey pox in humans to mouse pox—should attempt to coordinate their efforts and share their insights, and investigators of other viral pests might usefully compare notes too. Likewise, the development of the skills of genetic mapping and manipulation that might allow the creation of a functional virus from scratch should be integrated into the rest of a national strategy.

Beyond those immediate applications, we should think more expansively about what might be related fields in this area. As suggested by the chapters of this book, disciplines rather removed from virology and immunology may make a contribution to this effort and may themselves benefit in the exchange. Ethics, obviously, needs to be integrated here—and the hard thinking needs to be undertaken promptly, lest our technical competency at bioengineering, including the ability to build a functional virus from simple genetic building blocks, emerges so quickly that it renders the philosophizing moot. Environmentalism must be drawn in, as an enhanced understanding of global biodiversity may inform our policy judgments regarding retention of a unique microbe. What range of genetic variability actually exists in the microbial world, and how important is it to retain this particular virus as an exemplar of an important, rare breed?

Closer to home, research into medical facilitative technologies can provide pathways for improved understanding of variola. For example, the creation of transgenic mice, rabbits, or monkeys, possessing essential characteristics of the human immune system, may be an indispensable tool. They could provide the substrate for variola experiments, facilitating the development of new vaccines or antivirals that could not be adequately tested on human beings. Lacking a suitable animal model for preliminary screening of candidate pharmaceuticals, researchers would be unable to complete the sorts of testing that the U.S. Food and Drug Administration would ordinarily demand before licensing a new product. Support for those developmental efforts should be enhanced, to promote the less glamorous efforts that undergird long-term successes.

The United States, and the world more generally, need more BL-4 laboratory facilities, too, including both more space for advanced research and additional hospitalization suites for emergency treatment of infected individuals. These days, important research agendas must often compete for the scarce resource of adequate laboratory opportunities, and the cost to those research projects of delayed or foregone investigations is mounting. These supplementary facilities must be held to the highest safety and security standards applicable to variola work—the London and Birmingham accidents sound a cautionary note—and routine WHO inspections should be a regular feature. If any more tragic reminders were necessary, we should only recall that prior to global eradication of smallpox, a primary venue for the spread of the disease was hospitals: even health professionals, dedicated to resisting the disease, consistently failed to diagnose and treat it adequately or to protect the public from its proliferation.

In general, the nation's public health system needs to be revitalized. Years of diminished funding have led to an erosion of core capabilities that may be stressed in a bioterrorism emergency. The system must be more adept at gathering relevant disease data in a systematic, reliable way; communicating quickly and securely between all levels of health care professionals; and coordinating the resources of various tiers of federal, state, and local responses. In support of those capacities, reform of the often antiquated and balkanized state statutes on police powers is overdue: in too many instances, the existing procedures for quarantine, isolation, commandeering of hospital facilities, and so forth are piecemeal and stuck in the nineteenth century.

11. Support more international cooperation, especially with Vector

There are, of course, dangers in disseminating biological expertise. Every facility that acquires advanced equipment and materials, every individual who learns novel techniques and capabilities, represents a potential that might be

---

"turned to the dark side," providing assistance to rogue states or terrorist organizations.

But in this sector, the better technique for dealing with those apprehensions would be to open the research more broadly, to allow more participants to contribute their knowledge and, in a related sense, to be reassured that we are not proceeding with offensive military goals in mind. In return, we would also seek to impose safeguards on the locations where the research is conducted and upon the applications of the acquired knowledge.

Foremost in this regard is the Vector laboratory in Koltsovo, Russia, the most advanced research site in the former Soviet biological warfare apparatus. Vector now embodies both special dangers (the weapons expertise of its personnel, now perhaps vulnerable to recruitment and brain drain; the dilapidated condition of some installations, now perhaps vulnerable to lapses in physical security) and special opportunities (the possibility of converting the physical plant and the human capital to cutting-edge civilian applications).

American and other assistance and cooperation can make the difference. Partnering with Vector can be mutually profitable, as Westerners exploit the expertise (often available at lower costs) and world-class facilities, while infusing capital, management, and complementary scientific mastery that can protect the investment. Some of the contribution will initially have to be in the form of outright grants of aid, especially to improve the security and safety of the operations and to assist in the conversion to benign applications. But some of it, especially at subsequent stages, can be market driven, and can be expected to return a profit.

Variola research will never, by itself, be sufficient to carry more than a small percentage of the enterprise. But it can provide a concrete starting point, an illustration of the advantages of collaboration and intelligent pooling of resources, where American, Russian, and other researchers ought to be able to turn the Vector facilities to valuable civilian uses.

More generally, we need to recall that variola presents us, once again, with a global problem. Disease has never respected national borders, and in an era of long-range missiles, international terrorism, and frequent flyers, the virus cannot be segregated from any target community. We simply cannot return to the old formula, isolation by reerecting a cordon sanitaire around America or the developed world—any attempt to do so would be unacceptably expensive and doomed to failure. Since smallpox is precisely a worldwide dilemma, everyone should share in resolution of it.

12. Consider what to do the next time the question of deliberate extinction comes up

Each case, of course, is unique. Our attitudes may differ with the next virus, bacteria, or parasite that our concerted action is able to remove from the biosphere. The appropriate terms and conditions for retention or extermination may vary, depending on whether the possibility exists for a resurgence of the disease; whether the particular pathogen has been, or could be, used as a biological weapon; whether we still have, or might some day have, research or other uses for the creature; whether it more fully meets the biologists' traditional definition of life; whether there might be secret stocks, stashed away someplace; whether it is susceptible to being re-created artificially through step-by-step reconstruction of the genetic map; and the like.

But my own conclusion would largely transcend all that. I would be inclined to retain any such microbe, just in case we might need it some day and because it better expresses our humanity to preserve such species. Variola, in fact, may turn out to be both the first and the toughest case—if we are not willing to destroy this inhospitable little bug, then perhaps nothing else would ever fall to the executioner.

Our general conceptual approach to the conundrum, too, should be improved. In the case of smallpox, consideration was initially confined largely to the World Health Organization and a small cluster of national health bureaucracies and individual experts. There, the pro-extermination momentum was generated, with little careful consideration of countervailing arguments or interdisciplinary analyses. Only late in the process, almost after it was too late, did opposition surface. Gradually the issue of variola's ultimate fate attracted more attention, prompting an embarrassing series of delays in the WHO destruction schedule. Under the pressure of more contemplative analysis, additional resistance appeared, and some experts who had initially favored destruction abruptly changed their minds. Even at that stage, an editorial in *The Lancet*, a British medical journal and leading observer of the smallpox controversy, opined that "The debate so far has been unsatisfactory. Thus one might even recommend destruction because arguments for retention are so weak or recommend retention because arguments for destruction are so weak."[1]

Variola has thus managed, just barely, to dodge the autoclave several times. That sort of erratic deadline-setting and deadline-breaking is itself an indicator that we have not yet gotten our act together on this important question, and we need to be more systematic and careful in our approach to the next endangered pathogen. These are not strictly health issues, and they do not need to be resolved on a crash basis.

CONCLUSION

In the end, the inquiry into the future of variola may reveal as much about humans as a species as it does about the virus. How should we think about this noxious little creature, and what should we do to protect ourselves from it without debasing ourselves in the process? For at least three millennia, we have been fellow travelers on earth, and for most of that time smallpox was at an advantage. Now that it is within our power to decide the fate of the microbe, what standards and procedures should govern our decision making?

At the bottom line, I think we can do better than throw it away.

Notes

Chapter 1

1. The authoritative histories of smallpox and humankind's struggles against it are Frank Fenner, D. A. Henderson, Isao Arita, Zdenek Jezek, and Ivan D. Ladnyi, *Smallpox and Its Eradication* (Geneva: World Health Organization, 1988), and Donald R. Hopkins, *Princes and Peasants: Smallpox in History* (Chicago: University of Chicago Press, 1983). See also James Cross Giblin, *When Plague Strikes: The Black Death, Smallpox, AIDS* (New York: Harper Collins, 1995); Abbas M. Behbehani, *The Smallpox Story: In Words and Pictures* (Kansas City: University of Kansas Medical Center, 1988); and Joel N. Shurkin, *The Invisible Fire: The Story of Mankind's Victory over the Ancient Scourge of Smallpox* (New York: Putnam, 1979).

2. T. B. Macaulay, *The History of England from the Accession of James II* (London: J.M. Dent and Sons, 1848).

3. Hopkins, *Princes and Peasants*, 14–15 (describing the author's personal inspection of the mummy in 1979); and Fenner et al., *Smallpox and Its Eradication*, 210–11.

4. Nicolau Barquet and Pere Domingo, "Smallpox: The Triumph over the Most Terrible of the Ministers of Death," *Annals of Internal Medicine* 127 (October 15, 1997), 635, http://38.232.17.254/journals/annals/15oct97/smallpox, p. 3, visited December 17, 1999 (citing inter alia, Mary II of England in 1694, Emperor Higashiyama of Japan in 1709, and Peter II of Russia in 1730); Ed Regis, *Virus Ground Zero: Stalking the Killer Viruses with the Centers for Disease Control* (New York: Pocket Books, 1996), 63.

5. Hopkins, *Princes and Peasants*, 41.

6. Abbas M. Behbehani, "Smallpox," in ed. Joshua Lederberg, *Encyclopedia of Microbiology*, vol. 4 (San Diego: Academic Press, 1992), 34; Hopkins, *Princes and Peasants*, 8, 52; Giblin, *When Plague Strikes*, 65–66; Fenner et al., *Smallpox and Its Eradication*, 215.

7. Hopkins, *Princes and Peasants*, 206 (quoting Spanish friar Fray Toribio Motolinia).

8. Hopkins, *Princes and Peasants* 207; Giblin, *When Plague Strikes*, 67–71; E. Wagner Stearn and Allen E. Stearn, *The Effect of Smallpox on the Destiny of the Amerindian* (Boston: B. Humphries, 1945), 127.

9. Michael Radetsky, "Smallpox: A History of Its Rise and Fall," *Pediatric Infectious Disease Journal* 18, no. 2 (February 1999), 85.

10. Fenner et al., *Smallpox and Its Eradication*, 199.

11. But see Fenner et al., *Smallpox and Its Eradication*, 4 (declining to recognize *Variola intermedius* as a distinct entity).

12. Fenner et al., *Smallpox and Its Eradication*, 246.

13. Fenner et al., *Smallpox and Its Eradication*, 307–8 (summarizing general consensus on four conditions that constituted contraindications to vaccination: immune disorders, eczema, pregnancy, and disorders of the central nervous system). See also D. A. Henderson, "Variola and Vaccinia," in ed. J. Claude Bennett and Fred Plum, *Cecil Textbook of Medicine*, 20th ed. (Philadelphia: W.B. Saunders, 1996), 1767–68; D. A. Henderson, "Smallpox as a Biological Weapon: Medical and Public Health Management, Consensus Statement of the Working Group on Civilian Biodefense," *Journal of the American Medical Association* 281, no. 22 (June 9, 1999), 2127, 2134–35; Advisory Committee on Immunization Practices, "Vaccinia (Smallpox) Vaccine Recommendations of the Advisory Committee on Immunization Practices," *MMWR Reports and Recommendations* 50 (June 22, 2001), 1–25.

14. Hopkins, *Princes and Peasants*, 87, 89–90; Fenner et al., *Smallpox and Its Eradication*, 231–32, 272.

15. Hopkins, *Princes and Peasants*, 133, 154, 197–98; Fenner et al., *Smallpox and Its Eradication*, 315–63.

16. Fenner et al., *Smallpox and Its Eradication*, 175, 196.

17. Hopkins, *Princes and Peasants*, 293–94.

18. Hopkins, *Princes and Peasants*, 294.

19. Hopkins, *Princes and Peasants*, 98.

20. Fenner et al., *Smallpox and Its Eradication*, 175, 394–95, 516–17, 1345.

21. Quoted in Hopkins, *Princes and Peasants*, 310.

22. Fenner et al., *Smallpox and Its Eradication*, 172, 333–35, 389–91.

23. Fenner et al., *Smallpox and Its Eradication*, 370–87, 393–99, 1007–8.

24. Fenner et al., *Smallpox and Its Eradication*, 410–18, 422–25.

25. Fenner et al., *Smallpox and Its Eradication*, 421–592.

26. Hopkins, *Princes and Peasants*, 310; Fenner et al., *Smallpox and Its Eradication*, 532.

27. Fenner et al., *Smallpox and Its Eradication*, 1338–40.

28. Fenner et al., *Smallpox and Its Eradication*, 1268–70.

29. Fenner et al., *Smallpox and Its Eradication*, 1269–70; Henderson et al., "Variola and Vaccinia," 2132.

30. James LeDuc and John Becher, "Current Status of Smallpox Vaccine: Letter to the editor," *Emerging Infectious Diseases* 5, no. 4 (July–August 1999), 593; Laurie Garrett, "The Nightmare of Bioterrorism," *Foreign Affairs* 80, no. 1 (January/February 2001), 76, 77.

31. See D. A. Henderson, "Smallpox: Clinical and Epidemiologic Features," *Emerging Infectious Diseases* 5, no. 4 (July–August 1999), http://www.cdc.gov/ncidod/EID/vol5no4/henderson.htm, p. 2 ("U.S. national vaccine stocks are sufficient to immunize only 6 to 7 million persons. This amount is only marginally sufficient for emergency needs. Plans are now being made to expand this reserve. However, at least 36 months are required before large quantities can be produced.")

32. Judith Miller and Sheryl Gay Stolberg, "Attacks Led to Push for More Smallpox Vaccine," *New York Times*, October 22, 2001, A1.

33. Dana Hedgpeth, "BioReliance vs. Bioterrorism," *Washington Post*, August 24, 2000, E1.

34. "Bioterrorism Concerns Spark First Smallpox Vaccine Production in 30 Years," *CBW Chronicle* 3, no. 2 (December 2000), 1; J. Donald Millar, "Paradox in Prevention: Managing the Threat of Smallpox Bioterrorism," *PHPAB's Health Policy Focus* (February 2000), p. 2.

35. Miller and Stolberg, "Attacks Led to Push for More Smallpox Vaccine," A1.

36. Gina Kolata, "'Cure' for Bioterror May Be Worse Than the Disease," *New York Times*, October 22, 2001, B9; Susan Okie and Justin Gillis, "U.S. Mounts Smallpox Vaccine Push," *Washington Post*, October 28, 2001, A18.

37. D. A. Henderson et al., "Smallpox as a Biological Weapon," 2127, 2132; LeDuc and Becher, "Current Status of Smallpox Vaccine," 593 (only 675 doses of VIG are available, and administration of them has been suspended due to discoloration of unknown cause and effect; the U.S. Department of Defense has recently contracted for the production of additional supplies); Advisory Committee on Immunization Practices, "Vaccinia (Smallpox) Vaccine Recommendations," 1–25 (noting that VIG does not negate all the adverse side effects of vaccinia exposure, and carries some contraindications of its own).

38. World Health Organization, "WHO Fact Sheet on Smallpox," www.who

.int/emc/diseases/smallpox/factsheet, visited February 7, 2002; World Health Organization, "Statement WHO/16: World Health Organization Announces Updated Guidance on Smallpox Vaccination," October 2, 2001.

39. Shurkin, *The Invisible Fire*, 408–9.

Chapter 2

1. See generally Thomas A. Scott, "Virus Diseases," in *Concise Encyclopedia of Biology* (Berlin, N.Y.: Walter de Gruyter, 1996), 1244, 1245; George B. Johnson and Peter H. Raven, *Biology: Principles & Explorations* (Austin: Holt, Rinehart, and Winston, 1996), 461; B. Innes, "Viruses," in *Encyclopedia of the Life Sciences*, vol. 10 (Tarrytown, N.Y.: Marshall Cavendish Corp., 1996), 1398, 1399.

2. "Human Pox Viruses," www.mni.uwo.ca/Bio221a/virus3.html, visited December 17, 1999. (Epidermal growth factor is a hormone that stimulates cell proliferation.)

3. See Frank Fenner, D. A. Henderson, Isao Arita, Zdenek Jezek, and Ivan D. Ladnyi, *Smallpox and Its Eradication* (Geneva: World Health Organization, 1988), 86.

4. Innes, "Viruses," 1404. Rick Weiss, "Genetic Find Could Lead to Creation of Life from Scratch in Lab," *Washington Post*, December 10, 1999, A8.

5. Alton Biggs, Chris Kapicka, and Linda Lundgren, *Biology: The Dynamics of Life* (New York: Glencoe, 1995), 376–85; Johnson and Raven, *Biology: Principles & Explorations*, 203–9; Paul Berg and Maxine Singer, *Dealing with Genes: The Language of Heredity* (Mill Valley, Calif.: Blackwell Scientific Publications, 1992), 79–103.

6. Theodore Friedmann, "Overcoming the Obstacles to Gene Therapy," *Scientific American* (June 1997), 96; Michael Blaese, "Gene Therapy for Cancer," *Scientific American* (June 1997), 111.

7. Carol Kaesuk Yoon, "If It Walks and Moos Like a Cow, It's a Pharmaceutical Factory," *New York Times*, May 1, 2000, A20.

8. Matthew Meselson, "Averting the Hostile Exploitation of Biotechnology," *CBW Conventions Bulletin* 48 (June 2000), 16.

9. "Bioweapons Labs 'Could Unleash Forgotten Diseases,'" *Nature* 412 (August 2, 2001), 470.

10. John Pickrell, "Imperial College Fined over Hybrid Virus Risk," *Science* 293 (August 3, 2001), 779.

11. Robert F. Massung et al., "Potential Virulence Determinants in Terminal Regions of Variola Smallpox Virus Genome," *Nature* 366 (December 23–30, 1993), 748.

12. Committee on the Assessment of Future Scientific Needs for Live Variola Virus, Institute of Medicine (hereinafter, IOM), National Academy of Sciences, *Assessment of Future Scientific Needs for Live Variola Virus* (Washington, D.C.: National Academy Press, 1999), 62–63.

13. See Laurie Garrett, "The Return of Infectious Disease," *Foreign Affairs* 75, no. 1 (January/February 1996), 66, 76.

14. Charles Siebert, "Smallpox Is Dead, Long Live Smallpox," *New York Times Magazine,* August 21, 1994, 30, 33.

15. World Health Organization, "Overcoming Antimicrobial Resistance," World Health Report on Infectious Diseases (2000).

16. IOM, *Assessment of Future Scientific Needs,* 53; James LeDuc and John Becher, "Current Status of Smallpox Vaccine: Letter to the Editor," *Emerging Infectious Diseases* 5, no. 4 (July–August 1999), 593.

17. Richard Preston, "The Demon in the Freezer," *New Yorker* 75, no. 18 (July 12, 1999), 44, 56 (citing estimate provided by D. A. Henderson).

18. Quoted in "Smallpox: U.S. to Oppose Destruction of Last Samples," *American Health Line,* April 23, 1999.

19. Quoted in Laurie Garrett, *Betrayal of Trust: The Collapse of Global Public Health* (New York: Hyperion, 2000), 502.

20. Fenner et al., *Smallpox and Its Eradication,* 1341.

21. Graeme Laver and Elspeth Garman, "The Origin and Control of Pandemic Influenza," *Science* 293 (September 7, 2001), 1776. Gina Kolata, "Genetic Material of Virus from 1918 Flu Is Found," *New York Times,* March 21, 1997, A1.

22. Joel Breman and D. A. Henderson, "Poxvirus Dilemmas: Monkeypox, Smallpox, and Biologic Terrorism," *New England Journal of Medicine* 339, no. 8 (August 20, 1998), 556.

23. World Health Organization, "Monkeypox," Fact Sheet No. 161 (December 1997); Wendy Orent, "Killer Pox in the Congo," *Discover* 20, no. 10 (October 1999).

24. Quoted in Jon Cohen, "Is An Old Virus Up to New Tricks?" *Science* 277 (July 18, 1997), 5324.

25. IOM, *Assessment of Future Scientific Needs,* 64–65.

26. Anne Platt McGinn, "The Resurgence of Infectious Diseases," in ed. Rob DeSalle, *Epidemic! The World of Infectious Disease* (New York: New Press, 1999), 165.

27. "A World without Polio," http://www.unicef.org/polio/abouteradication.htm, visited February 26, 2002.

28. World Health Organization, "Dracunculiasis: The Disease," www.who.int/ctd/dracun/disease, visited November 2, 2000.

Chapter 3

1. Regarding the history of biological weapons generally, and smallpox in particular, see Charles C. Flowerree, "Chemical and Biological Weapons and Arms Control," in ed. Richard Dean Burns, *Encyclopedia of Arms Control*, vol. 1 (New York: Scribner's, 1993), 999; John Ellis van Courtland Moon, "Controlling Chemical and Biological Weapons through World War II," in ed. Richard Dean Burns, *Encyclopedia of Arms Control*, vol. 1 (New York: Scribner's, 1993), 657; Erhard Geissler and John Ellis van Courtland Moon (eds.), *Biological and Toxin Weapons: Research, Development and Use from the Middle Ages to 1945* (New York: Oxford University Press, 1999); Jonathan B. Tucker, ed., *Toxic Terror: Assessing Terrorist Use of Chemical and Biological Weapons* (Cambridge, Mass.: MIT Press, 2000); Erhard Geissler, ed., *Biological and Toxin Weapons Today* (New York: Oxford University Press, 1986); Erhard Geissler and John P. Woodall, eds., *Control of Dual-Threat Agents: The Vaccines for Peace Programme* (New York: Oxford University Press, 1994); Leonard A. Cole, *The Eleventh Plague: The Politics of Biological and Chemical Warfare* (New York: W.H. Freeman, 1997); Charles Piller and Keith R. Yamamoto, *Gene Wars: Military Control over the New Genetic Technologies* (New York: Beech Tree Books, 1988); John Parker, *The Killing Factory: The Top Secret World of Germ and Chemical Warfare* (London: Smith Gryphon, 1996); Susan Wright, *Preventing a Biological Arms Race* (Cambridge, Mass.: MIT Press, 1990).

2. Paul E. Steiner, *Disease in the Civil War: Natural Biological Warfare in 1861–1865* (Springfield, Ill.: C.C. Thomas, 1968).

3. Alberico Gentili, *The Law of War*, book 2, chapter 6 (1598), reprinted in *The Classics of International Law*, vol. 2, no. 16 (Buffalo, N.Y.: William S. Hein, 1995) (John C. Rolfe, translator; James Brown Scott, editor), 155.

4. Hugo Grotius, *De Jure Belli Ac Pacis*, book 3, chapter 15 (1625), reprinted in *The Classics of International Law*, vol. 2, no. 3 (Buffalo, N.Y.: William S. Hein, 1995) (Francis W. Kelsey, translator; James Brown Scott, editor), 652.

5. Emmerich de Vattel, *The Law of Nations*, book 3, chapter 8, sec. 156 (1758), (new ed., ed. Joseph Chittey, Philadelphia: T. and J.W. Johnson, 1883), 361.

6. Francis Parkman, *The Conspiracy of Pontiac* (1851; reprinted New York: Literary Classics of the United States, 1991), 646–49; Bernhard Knollenberg, "General Amherst and Germ Warfare," *Mississippi Valley Historical Review* (December 1954), 489–94; James A. Poupard, Linda A. Miller, and Lindsay Granshaw, "The Use of Smallpox as a Biological Weapon in the French and Indian War of 1763," *ASM News* 55, no. 3 (1989), 122.

7. See Poupard, Miller, and Granshaw, "The Use of Smallpox as a Biological Weapon," 123, suggesting that Bouquet may have drawn a blank line in his letter,

instead of naming the particular tribe that was to be the target of the plot, as a crude measure of "operational security," to maintain the secrecy of the activity.

8. Parkman, *The Conspiracy of Pontiac*, 646–49; Knollenberg, "General Amherst and Germ Warfare," 489–94; Poupard, Miller, and Granshaw, "The Use of Smallpox as a Biological Weapon," 122.

9. Poupard, Miller, and Granshaw, "The Use of Smallpox as a Biological Weapon," 124, quoting E. Wagner Stearn and Allen E. Stearn, *The Effect of Smallpox on the Destiny of the Amerindian* (Boston: B. Humphries, 1945).

10. Elizabeth A. Fenn, *Pox Americana: The Great Smallpox Epidemic of 1775–82* (New York: Hill and Wang, 2001), 50, 62, 89.

11. "Instructions for the Government of Armies of the United States in the Field (Lieber Code), promulgated as General Orders 100, 1863," reprinted in M. Cherif Bassiouni, ed., *A Manual on International Humanitarian Law and Arms Control Agreements* (New York: Transnational Publishers, 2000), 273, article 70.

12. Parker, *The Killing Factory*, 18–26; Moon, "Controlling Chemical and Biological Weapons," 663.

13. *Geneva Protocol for the Prohibition of the Use in War of Asphyxiating, Poisonous or other Gases, and of Bacteriological Methods of Warfare*, 26 UNTS 571, TIAS No. 8061, June 17, 1925.

14. Barton J. Bernstein, "America's Biological Warfare Program in the Second World War," *Journal of Strategic Studies* (September 1988), 292.

15. Bernstein, "America's Biological Warfare Program," 298, 304.

16. Erhard Geissler, "Biological Warfare Activities in Germany, 1923–45," in Geissler and Moon, *Biological and Toxin Weapons*, 91, 121.

17. See generally Peter Williams and David Wallace, *Unit 731: Japan's Secret Biological Warfare in World War II* (New York: Free Press, 1989); Sheldon Harris, "The Japanese Biological Warfare Programme: An Overview," in Geissler and Moon, *Biological and Toxin Weapons*, 127–52.

18. Jean Pascal Zanders and Maria Wahlberg, "Chemical and Biological Weapon Developments and Arms Control," in *SIPRI Yearbook 2000: Armaments, Disarmament, and International Security* (Stockholm: Almquist & Wiksell; New York: Humanities Press, 2000), 509, 514–16.

19. Estimate by Stockholm International Peace Research Institute, cited in Eileen Choffnes, "The Environmental Legacy of Biological Weapons Testing," in ed. Lakshman D. Guruswamy and Susan R. Grillot, *Arms Control and the Environment* (Ardsley, N.Y.: Transnational Publishers, 2001), 159, 164, note 4.

20. Parker, *The Killing Factory*, 121.

21. Bill Patrick, quoted in Shannon Brownlee, "Clear and Present Danger," *Washington Post Magazine*, October 28, 2001, 8, 21.

22. Senate Select Committee to Study Government Operations with Respect to Intelligence, *Unauthorized Storage of Toxic Agents*, 94th Congress, 1st sess., September 16–18, 1975 (testimony of CIA Director William Colby and Nathan Gordon).

23. See generally Ken Alibek, with Stephen Handelman, *Biohazard* (New York: Random House, 1999).

24. Alibek, *Biohazard*, 43; Jonathan B. Tucker, "Biological Weapons in the Former Soviet Union: An Interview with Dr. Kenneth Alibek," *Nonproliferation Review* 6, no. 3 (spring–summer 1999), 1.

25. See Howard Witt, "Russian Lab Sits on Dread Secret: Smallpox Cache; Fears of Terrorists' Stealing Virus," *Arizona Republic*, February 10, 1994.

26. Ken Alibek, "Behind the Mask: Biological Warfare," *Perspective* 9, no. 1 (September–October 1998).

27. Wendy Orent, "The End of the Trail for Smallpox?" *Los Angeles Times*, August 2, 1998, M2.

28. Oliver Thranert, "Strengthening the Biological Weapons Convention: An Urgent Task," *Contemporary Security Policy* 17, no. 3 (December 1996), 347, 359.

29. Amy E. Smithson, "Separating Fact from Fiction: The Australia Group and the Chemical Weapons Convention," Henry L. Stimson Center, Occasional Paper No. 34 (March 1997).

30. Ron Purver, "Chemical and Biological Terrorism: The Threat According to the Open Literature," *Canadian Security Intelligence Service* (June 1995), 3.

31. Quoted in Graham S. Pearson, "Deliberate Disease: Why Biological Warfare is a Real Concern," International Security Information Service, Briefing Paper No. 6, (July 1996), 5.

32. *Convention on the Prohibition of the Development, Production and Stockpiling of Bacteriological (Biological) and Toxin Weapons and on Their Destruction* (hereinafter, *BWC*), signed at Washington, London, and Moscow, April 10, 1972, art. I.

33. *BWC*, art. I, para. 1.

34. *BWC*, art. I, para. 1.

35. Jeanne Guillemin, *Anthrax: The Investigation of a Deadly Outbreak* (Berkeley: University of California Press, 1999).

36. Jonathan B. Tucker, "The 'Yellow Rain' Controversy: Lessons for Arms Control Compliance," *Nonproliferation Review* 8, no. 1 (spring 2001), 25; Sterling Seagrave, *Yellow Rain: A Journey through Terror* (New York: M. Evans, 1981); Thomas D. Seeley, Joan W. Nowicke, Matthew Meselson, Jeanne Guillemin, and Pongthep Akratanakul, "Yellow Rain," *Scientific American* (September 1985), 128.

37. Center for Civilian Biodefense Studies, "Smallpox," www.hopkins-biodefense.org/pages/agents/agentsmallpox, visited November 12, 2001.

38. U.S. General Accounting Office, "Biological Weapons: Effort to Reduce Former Soviet Threat Offers Benefits, Poses New Risks," GAO/NSIAD-00-138 (April 2000), 28.

39. Howard L. Rosenberg, "Russia's Smallpox Stash," March 18, 1999, abcnews.de.onair/2020/2020_990317_smallpox_feature2, visited February 29, 2000 (describing Vector's once-gleaming viral research apparatus as "a half-empty facility protected by a handful of guards who had not been paid for months").

40. Judith Miller, "U.S. Helps Russia Turn Germ Center to Peace Uses," *New York Times,* January 8, 2000, A3; Anthony Rimmington, "From Military to Industrial Complex? The Conversion of Biological Weapons' Facilities in the Russian Federation," *Contemporary Security Policy* 17, no. 1 (April 1996), 80.

41. Executive Order 12938 (November 14, 1994), pursuant to International Emergency Economic Powers Act, 50 U.S.C.A. *(U.S. Code Annotated)* 1701 et seq., renewed annually, most recently on November 9, 2000. Penalties for assisting a foreign state in acquiring weapons of mass destruction were increased in 1998.

42. Javed Ali, "Chemical Weapons and the Iran-Iraq War: A Case Study in Noncompliance," *Nonproliferation Review* 8, no. 1 (spring 2001), 43; Flowerree, "Chemical and Biological Weapons," 1002.

43. U.S. Government, Counterproliferation Program Review Committee, "Report on Activities and Programs for Countering Proliferation and NBC Terrorism" (May 1998), 3.11–12; Pearson, "Deliberate Disease," 5.

44. Central Intelligence Agency, "Unclassified Report to Congress on the Acquisition of Technology Relating to Weapons of Mass Destruction and Advanced Conventional Munitions, 1 July Through 31 December 2000" (September 2001); U.S. Department of Defense, "Chemical and Biological Defense Program," Annual Report to Congress, July 2001.

45. John R. Bolton, "Remarks to the Fifth Biological Weapons Convention Review Conference Meeting," November 19, 2001, www.state.gov/t/us/rm/2001/aug_nov/index, visited January 18, 2002.

46. William J. Broad and Judith Miller, "Government Report Says 3 Nations Hide Stocks of Smallpox," *New York Times,* June 13, 1999, A1; David Brown, "Destruction of Smallpox Samples is Reassessed," *Washington Post,* March 15, 1999, A1.

47. Judith Miller and William J. Broad, "Bio Weapons in Mind, Iranians Lure Needy Ex-Soviet Scientists," *New York Times,* December 8, 1998, A1; Tucker, "Biological Weapons in the Former Soviet Union," 1, 5.

48. Erhard Geissler, "Arms Control, Health Care and Technology Transfer under the Vaccines for Peace Programme," in Geissler and Woodall, *Control of Dual-Threat Agents,* 10, 22; Robert Chandler, "U.S. Strategists Must Prepare for

Growing Biological Threat," *Defense News,* November 11–17, 1996; Cole, *The Eleventh Plague,* 4, 7–8 (citing arms control expert Kathleen Bailey).

49. Jody Warrick and Steve Fainaru, "Bioterrorism Preparations Lacking at Lowest Level," *Washington Post,* October 22, 2001, A7; Ceci Connolly, "U.S. Officials Reorganize Strategy on Bioterrorism," *Washington Post,* November 8, 2001, A1.

50. Ceci Connolly, "Bush Promotes Plans to Fight Bioterrorism," *Washington Post,* February 6, 2002, A3.

51. "U.S. Called Vulnerable to Biological Attack," *Washington Post,* July 24, 2001, A5.

52. "Dark Winter," overview at www.homelandsecurity.org/darkwinter, visited December 27, 2001.

53. Quoted in Susan Okie and Justin Gillis, "U.S. Mounts Smallpox Vaccine Push," *Washington Post,* October 28, 2001, A18.

54. Judith Miller, "U.S. Set to Retain Smallpox Stocks," *New York Times,* November 16, 2001, A1; David Brown, "U.S. Wants the Smallpox Virus Preserved for Further Research," *Washington Post,* November 17, 2001, A9.

55. Rick Weiss, "Ordering Germs? There Are Hurdles First," *Washington Post,* October 12, 2001, A27.

56. *United States v Harris,* 961 FSupp 1127 (SD Ohio 1997); Jessica Eve Stern, "Larry Wayne Harris (1998)," in Tucker, *Toxic Terror,* 227.

57. Quoted in William J. Broad, "Smaller, Cheaper, Stealthier, Deadlier," *New York Times,* February 11, 2001, 18.

58. Quoted in William J. Broad, "Experts Call for Better Assessment of Threats," *New York Times,* October 2, 2001, D1.

59. Susan Wright, "Biowar Treaty in Danger," *Bulletin of the Atomic Scientists* 47, no. 7 (September 1991), 36.

Chapter 4

1. See generally David Hunter, James Salzman, and Durwood Zaelke, *International Environmental Law and Policy* (New York: Foundation Press, 1998); Lakshman Guruswamy and Brent Hendricks, *International Environmental Law in a Nutshell* (St. Paul, Minn.: West Publishing, 1997); Marjorie L. Reaka-Kudla, Don E. Wilson, and Edward O. Wilson, eds., *Biodiversity II* (Washington, D.C.: Joseph Henry Press, 1997); Edward O. Wilson, *The Diversity of Life* (Cambridge, Mass.: Belknap Press of Harvard University Press, 1992); Paul Ehrlich and Anne Ehrlich, *Extinction: The Causes and Consequences of the Disappearance of Species* (New York: Random House, 1981).

2. William H. Rogers Jr., *Environmental Law,* 2d ed. (St. Paul, Minn.: West Publishing, 1994); Robert L. Fischman and Mark S. Squillace, *Environmental Decisionmaking,* 3d ed. (Cincinnati, Ohio: Anderson Publishing, 2000); Andy Purvis and Andy Hector, "Getting the Measure of Biodiversity," *Nature* 405 (May 11, 2000), 212; Jon Hutton and Barnabas Dickson, eds., *Endangered Species, Threatened Convention: The Past, Present and Future of CITES* (London: Earthscan: 2000); Bryan G. Norton, ed., *The Preservation of Species: The Value of Biological Diversity* (Princeton, N.J.: Princeton University Press, 1986); Niles Eldredge, *The Miner's Canary: Unraveling the Mysteries of Extinction* (New York: Prentice Hall, 1991).

3. Hunter, Salzman, and Zaelke, *International Environmental Law and Policy,* 1518.

4. United Nations, *Stockholm Declaration of the United Nations Conference on the Human Environment* (hereinafter, *Stockholm Declaration*), adopted June 16, 1972, UN Doc. A/CONF.48/14/Rev. 1 at 3 (1973), 11 ILM 1416 (1972), proclamation 2.

5. Wilson, *The Diversity of Life,* 132–33; Timothy Swanson, *Global Action for Diversity: An International Framework for Implementing the Convention on Biological Diversity* (London: Earthscan, 1997).

6. Swanson, *Global Action for Diversity,* 8, 21; Wilson, *The Diversity of Life,* 134–39.

7. Wilson, *The Diversity of Life,* 133–35; Swanson, *Global Action for Diversity,* 8.

8. Purvis and Hector, "Getting the Measure of Biodiversity," 212, 213.

9. Wilson, *The Diversity of Life,* 260–72; Guruswamy and Hendricks, *International Environmental Law in a Nutshell,* 86–87.

10. Wilson, *The Diversity of Life,* 280; Ehrlich and Ehrlich, *Extinction,* 8; Timothy M. Swanson, *The International Regulation of Extinction* (Washington Square: New York University Press, 1994), 51.

11. Hunter, Salzman, and Zaelke, *International Environmental Law and Policy,* 944–45; Charles C. Mann and Mark L. Plummer, *Noah's Choice: The Future of Endangered Species* (New York: Knopf, 1996).

12. Hunter, Salzman, and Zaelke, *International Environmental Law and Policy,* 5–6, 939–44; Robert Costanza et al., "The Value of the World's Ecosystems and Natural Capital," *Nature* 387 (1997), 253.

13. Hunter, Salzman, and Zaelke, *International Environmental Law and Policy,* 940; Swanson, *Global Action for Diversity,* 64.

14. See Rogers, *Environmental Law,* 995.

15. *Convention on Biological Diversity* (hereinafter, *Biodiversity Convention*), 31 I.L.M. 818, signed June 5, 1992, entered into force December 29, 1993, arts. 5, 7, 8, 9. See also art. 6, calling for conservation by each party "in accordance with its particular conditions and circumstances."

16. *Biodiversity Convention,* preamble, para. 1.

17. *Biodiversity Convention,* art. 20.2.

18. *Biodiversity Convention,* art. 2.

19. *Biodiversity Convention,* art. 6.

20. *Biodiversity Convention,* art. 9.

21. *Convention on Nature Protection and Wildlife Preservation in the Western Hemisphere* (hereinafter, *Western Convention*), October 12, 1940, preamble, para. 1.

22. *Western Convention,* art. VIII.

23. *African Convention on the Conservation of Nature and Natural Resources* (hereinafter, *African Convention*), September 15, 1968, art. II, preamble, para. 1.

24. *African Convention,* art. XVII.1(3).

25. See Hunter, Salzman, and Zaelke, *International Environmental Law and Policy,* 939, 1035.

26. *Convention on International Trade in Endangered Species of Wild Fauna and Flora* (hereinafter, *CITES*), March 3, 1973, preamble, para. 3.

27. *CITES,* art. III.2(a), IV2(a), V.

28. *CITES,* art. VIII.6.

29. *Stockholm Declaration,* Principles 1–4.

30. United Nations General Assembly, *World Charter for Nature,* adopted October 28, 1982, G.A. Res. 37/7 (Annex), UN GAOR, 37th Sess., Supp. No. 51, at 17, UN Doc. A/37/51, 22 I.L.M. 455 (1983), preamble, para. 3, arts. I.2. II.10.

31. *Final Act of the Conference on Security and Co-operation in Europe,* adopted at Helsinki, August 1, 1975, 14 I.L.M. 1292.

32. *Stockholm Declaration,* Principle 21. See Hunter, Salzman, and Zaelke, *International Environmental Law and Policy,* 287–88 (emphasizing importance of Principle 21).

33. United Nations Conference on Environment and Development, *Rio Declaration on Environment and Development* (hereinafter, *Rio Declaration*), adopted Rio de Janeiro, June 13, 1992, UN Doc. A/Conf.151/26, 31 I.L.M. 874, Principles 1, 2, 4. See generally Hunter, Salzman, and Zaelke, *International Environmental Law and Policy,* 98–104.

34. *Stockholm Declaration,* preamble, para. 5.

35. *Rio Declaration,* Principle 17.

36. *Biodiversity Convention,* art. 2.

37. United Nations Conference on Environment and Development, *Agenda 21,* adopted at Rio de Janeiro, June 13, 1992, UN Doc. A/CONF 151/26, Chapter 15.3.

38. *Rio Declaration,* Principle 15.

39. *Stockholm Declaration,* proclamation 1.

40. 16 U.S.C.A. *(U.S. Code Annotated),* 4321, 4331.

41. 16 U.S.C.A. 4431 (b)(4).

42. 42 U.S.C.A. 4332 (C)(v).

43. 16 U.S.C.A. 1531.

44. *Tennessee Valley Authority v Hill*, 437 U.S. 153, 184, 187, 98 SCt 2279, 2297, 57 LEd 117 (1978).

45. 16 U.S.C.A. 1532 (8) (the definition further extends to cover "any part, product, egg, or offspring thereof, of the dead body or parts thereof").

46. 16 U.S.C.A. 1532 (14).

47. 16 U.S.C.A. 1532 (16). ("The term 'species' includes any subspecies of fish or wildlife or plants, and any distinct population segment of any species of vertebrate fish or wildlife which interbreeds when mature.")

48. 16 U.S.C.A. 1532 (6).

49. *Tennessee Valley Authority v Hill*, 437 U.S. 153, 178, 98 SCt 2279, 57 LEd 117 (1978) (quoting House report).

50. Wilson, *The Diversity of Life*, 351.

Chapter 5

1. Many of the documents used in the preparation of this chapter are official publications of the World Health Organization—its organic instruments, resolutions of its organs, reports of its committees, and so on. Most of them are available through the organization's Website and are not separately cited here. See also Giuseppe Schiavone, *International Organizations: A Directory and Dictionary*, 3d ed. (New York: St. Martin's, 1993); Robert N. Wells Jr., ed., *Peace by Pieces: United Nations Agencies and Their Roles* (Metuchen, N.J.: Scarecrow, 1991); *Worldmark Encyclopedia of the Nations: The United Nations*, vol. 1, 10th ed. (New York: Gale Research, 2001); *Toward Mankind's Better Health, Oceana Publications, Study Guide Series*, vol. 3 (Dobbs Ferry, N.Y.: Oceana Publications, 1963); Allyn L. Taylor, "Controlling the Global Spread of Infectious Diseases: Toward a Reinforced Role for the International Health Regulations," *Houston Law Review* 33 (1997), 1327; David P. Fidler, "The Future of the World Health Organization: What Role for International Law?" *Vanderbilt Journal of Transnational Law* 31, no. 5 (November 1998), 1079; David P. Fidler, *International Law and Infectious Diseases* (New York: Oxford University Press, 1999); Paul F. Basch, *Textbook of International Health*, 2d ed. (New York: Oxford University Press, 1999); World Health Organization, *The First Ten Years of the World Health Organization* (Geneva: World Health Organization, 1958); Javed Siddiqi, *World Health and World Politics: The World Health Organization and the UN System* (Columbia, S.C.: University of South Carolina Press, 1995); Yves Beigbeder, *The World Health Organization* (Boston: M. Nijhoff, 1998).

2. World Health Organization, *Constitution of the World Health Organization,* opened for signature in New York July 22, 1946, 62 Stat. 2679, 14 UNTS 185, preamble. See also World Health Organization, "Mission Statement," www.who.int/aboutwho/en/mission.htm, visited December 8, 2000.

3. World Health Organization, "Policy and Budget for One WHO," 11–15, and "Overview of Expenditure Plans," 11, both at www.who.int; World Health Organization, "What is the budget of the WHO?" www.who.int/aboutwho/en/qa6.htm, visited December 8, 2000.

4. World Health Organization, "About WHO: Rapid Overview," www.who.int/aboutwho/en/rapid.htm, visited December 8, 2000; World Health Organization, "Regulations for Study and Scientific Groups, Collaborating Institutions and Other Mechanisms of Collaboration," www.policy.who.int/cgi-bin.

5. *Worldmark Encyclopedia,* 252–53; *Toward Mankind's Better Health,* 24–25, 46–51; World Health Organization, "Regulations for Study and Scientific Groups"; World Health Organization, "Regulations for Expert Advisory Panels and Committees," reprinted in World Health Organization, *Basic Documents,* 43d ed. (Geneva: WHO, 2001), 101–9.

6. Siddiqi, *World Health and World Politics,* 82–100; U.S. Central Intelligence Agency, "The Global Infectious Disease Threat and Its Implications for the United States," National Intelligence Estimate 99-17D (January 2000), 16.

7. Allyn Lise Taylor, "Making the World Health Organization Work: A Legal Framework for Universal Access to the Conditions for Health," *American Journal of Law & Medicine* 18, no. 4 (1992), 301, 302–3, 339–43.

8. Fidler, "The Future of the World Health Organization," 1079. See also David P. Fidler, "Return of the Fourth Horseman: Emerging Infectious Diseases and International Law," *Minnesota Law Review* 81, no. 4 (April 1997), 771.

9. World Health Assembly, *Resolution WHA 33.4: Global Smallpox Eradication,* May 14, 1980.

10. "Memoranda: Destruction of Variola Virus: Memorandum from a WHO Meeting," Bulletin of the World Health Organization 72, no. 6 (1994), 841, 842–43.

11. World Health Organization, Department of Communicable Disease Surveillance and Response, "Report of the meeting of the Ad Hoc Committee on Orthopoxvirus Infections," Geneva, Switzerland, January 14–15, 1999, WHO/CDS/CSR/99.1.

12. World Health Organization, Department of Communicable Disease Surveillance and Response, "WHO Advisory Committee on Variola Virus Research: Report of a WHO Meeting, Geneva, Switzerland, 6–9 December 1999" (hereinafter, "WHO Advisory Committee"), WHO/CDS/CSR/2000.1; World Health

Organization, "Report by the Secretariat, Smallpox Eradication: Destruction of Variola Virus Stocks," April 10, 2000, EB 106/3.

13. World Health Assembly, *Resolution 55.15,* May 18, 2002.

14. "WHO Advisory Committee," 3.

15. "WHO Advisory Committee," 2.

16. World Health Organization, "Report by the Secretariat, Smallpox Eradication: Temporary Retention of Variola Virus Stocks," A54/16, April 11, 2001, 2.

17. World Health Organization, "Report by the Secretariat, Smallpox Eradication: Destruction of Variola Virus Stocks," EB109/17, December 20, 2001, para. 10, 18.

18. World Health Organization, "Report by the Secretariat, Smallpox Eradication: Destruction of Variola Virus Stocks," EB109/17, December 20, 2001, para. 10, 18.

19. David Brown, "Biological, Chemical Threat Is Termed Tricky, Complex," *Washington Post,* September 30, 2001, A12 (quoting C. J. Peters, a medical virologist at the University of Texas, Galveston, and former branch chief at the Centers for Disease Control).

20. Quoted in Lawrence K. Altman, "Lab Samples of Smallpox Win Reprieve," *New York Times,* January 19, 1995, A15.

21. Susan Okie, "US to Oppose Destroying Smallpox Stocks," *Washington Post,* April 23, 1999, A2; Judith Miller and Lawrence K. Altman, "Health Panel Recommends a Reprieve for Smallpox," *New York Times,* May 22, 1999, A3.

22. Wendy Orent, "The Smallpox Wars: Biowarfare vs. Public Health," *American Prospect* 44 (May–June 1999), 49, 53.

23. D. A. Henderson, "Deliberations Regarding the Destruction of Smallpox Virus: A Historical Overview, 1980–1998." Working paper for meeting of a Committee of the Institute of Medicine (November 20, 1998).

24. Ken Alibek and Stephen Handelman, "Smallpox Could Still Be a Danger," *New York Times,* May 24, 1999, A27 (arguing that "The only reliable protection for sensitive smallpox work is a truly transparent regime" in which "scientists from all countries could work together under the scrutiny of the international community"); Lev S. Sandakhchiev, "We'd Better Think Twice Before Eradicating All Smallpox Virus Stocks," *The Scientist* 7, no. 16 (August 23, 1993), 11.

Chapter 6

1. G. MacMunn, *The Underworld of India* (1933), 233, quoted in Donald R. Hopkins, *Princes and Peasants: Smallpox in History* (Chicago: University of Chicago Press: 1983), 163.

2. S. O. Fadeyi, "Yoruba Beliefs Regarding Smallpox Prevention and Folklore,"

in *Handbook for Smallpox Eradication Programmes in Endemic Areas* (World Health Organization, 1967), V-20, quoted in Hopkins, *Princes and Peasants*, 202.

3. Hopkins, *Princes and Peasants*, 100–102.

4. Bernard E. Rollin, *The Frankenstein Syndrome: Ethical and Social Issues in the Genetic Engineering of Animals* (New York: Cambridge University Press, 1995), 109.

5. Jonathan Schell, *The Fate of the Earth* (New York: Knopf, 1982), 115. Schell refers to species extermination as a "second death," or as "the death of death," because it totally eliminates the possibility of any future lives for our potential successors (119).

6. Otar Andzhaparidze, quoted in Charles Siebert, "Smallpox Is Dead, Long Live Smallpox," *New York Times Magazine*, August 21, 1994, 30, 32.

7. Quoted in Richard Preston, "The Demon in the Freezer," *New Yorker* 75, no. 18 (July 12, 1999), 44, 52.

8. David Ehrenfeld, *The Arrogance of Humanism* (New York: Oxford University Press, 1978), 207–8 (emphasis omitted).

9. *Convention on the Prohibition of the Development, Production and Stockpiling of Bacteriological (Biological) and Toxin Weapons and on Their Destruction*, signed at Washington, London, and Moscow, April 10, 1972, 26 U.S.T. 583, 1015 U.N.T.S. 163, 11 I.L.M. 309, art. I.

10. Quoted in Siebert, "Smallpox Is Dead," 32.

11. Christopher Stone, "Should Trees Have Standing: Toward Legal Rights for Natural Objects," *Southern California Law Review* 45 (1972), 450, reprinted in Christopher D. Stone, *Should Trees Have Standing and Other Essays on Law, Morals, and the Environment* (Dobbs Ferry, N.Y.: Oceana Publications, 1996), 1.

Chapter 7

1. Among the leading literature sources presenting the arguments, sometimes vociferously, for or against eradication of variola, are Brian W. J. Mahy, Jeffrey W. Almond, Kenneth I. Berns, Robert M. Chanock, Dmitry K. Lvov, Ralf K. Petterson, Herman G. Schatzmeyer, and Frank Fenner, "The Remaining Stocks of Smallpox Should Be Destroyed," *Science* 262, no. 5137 (November 19, 1993); Wolfgang K. Joklik, Bernard Moss, Bernard N. Fields, David L. Bishop, and Lev S. Sandakhchiev, "Why the Smallpox Virus Stocks Should Not Be Destroyed," *Science* 262, no. 5137 (November 19, 1993); Karen Young Kreeger, "Smallpox Extermination Proposal Stirs Scientists," *The Scientist* 8, no. 22 (November 14, 1994), 1; Jeffrey Fox, "WHO Assembly to Consider Smallpox Destruction," *ASM News* 60, no. 4 (1994), 183; Lawrence K. Altman, "Fate of a Virus: A Special Report," *New York Times*, August

30, 1993, A1; Bernard Roizman, Wolfgang Joklik, Bernard Fields, and Bernard Moss, "The Destruction of Smallpox Virus Stocks in National Repositories: A Grave Mistake and a Bad Precedent," *Infectious Agents and Disease* 3, no. 5 (1994), 215; Center for Security Policy, "A Pox on *Our* House: Will Clinton's NSC Compound America's Vulnerability to Biological Warfare?" Decision Brief No. 99-D 36 (March 17, 1999); Walter R. Dowdle, "Destruction of the Smallpox Virus: Why the Debate?" *Clinical Microbiology Newsletter* 17, no. 13 (1995), 101; Charles Siebert, "Smallpox Is Dead, Long Live Smallpox," *New York Times Magazine,* August 21, 1994, 30.

2. James Brooke, "Military Pilot Went Down with Plane, Air Force Says," *New York Times,* April 26, 1997, 8. By coincidence, the newspapers on that same day also featured reports about a civilian tractor-trailer driver who somehow stole four U.S. Air Force air-to-ground training missiles and hid them in a building supply store for three days and about U.S. Army officials losing track of another truck that was carrying mortars and machine guns to California. Sam Howe Verhovek, "After Searching, Air Force Finds 4 Training Missiles," *New York Times,* April 26, 1997, 8. More recently, a Connecticut nuclear power plant has admitted that it lost track of two spent nuclear fuel rods. David M. Herszenhorn, "A Sheepish Search for Missing Fuel Rods," *New York Times,* January 8, 2001, A17.

Chapter 9

1. "Another Reprieve for Smallpox Virus (editorial)," *The Lancet* 342, no. 8870 (August 28, 1993), 505.

Select Bibliography

Books and Book Chapters

Alibek, Ken, with Handelman, Stephen. *Biohazard*. New York: Random House, 1999.

American Law Institute. *Restatement (Third) of the Foreign Relations Law of the United States*. Philadelphia: American Law Institute, 1986.

Basch, Paul F. *Textbook of International Health*, 2d ed. New York: Oxford University Press, 1999.

Bassiouni, M. Cherif, ed. *A Manual on International Humanitarian Law and Arms Control Agreements*. New York: Transnational Publishers, 2000.

Beauchamp, Tom, and Childress, James. *Principles of Biomedical Ethics*, 4th ed. New York: Oxford University Press, 1994.

Behbehani, Abbas M. "Smallpox." In ed. Joshua Lederberg, *Encyclopedia of Microbiology*, vol. 4. San Diego: Academic Press, 1992, 34.

———. *The Smallpox Story: In Words and Pictures*. Kansas City: University of Kansas Medical Center, 1988.

Beigbeder, Yves. *The World Health Organization*. Boston: M. Nijhoff, 1998.

Bekoff, Marc, ed. *Encyclopedia of Animal Rights and Animal Welfare*. Westport, Conn.: Greenwood Press, 1998.

Berg, Paul, and Singer, Maxine. *Dealing with Genes: The Language of Heredity*. Mill Valley, Calif.: Blackwell Scientific Publications, 1992.

Biggs, Alton, Kapicka, Chris, and Lundgren, Linda. *Biology: The Dynamics of Life*. New York: Glencoe, 1995.

Bilderbeek, Simone. *Biodiversity and International Law: The Effectiveness of International Environmental Law.* Washington, D.C.: IOS Press, 1992.

Bruce, Donald, and Bruce, Ann, eds. *Engineering Genesis: The Ethics of Genetic Engineering in Non-Human Species.* London: Earthscan, 1998.

Choffnes, Eileen. "The Environmental Legacy of Biological Weapons Testing." In ed. Lakshman D. Guruswamy and Susan R. Grillot, *Arms Control and the Environment.* Ardsley, N.Y.: Transnational Publishers, 2001.

Cole, Leonard A. *The Eleventh Plague: The Politics of Biological and Chemical Warfare.* New York: W.H. Freeman, 1997.

Committee on the Assessment of Future Scientific Needs for Live Variola Virus, Institute of Medicine, National Academy of Sciences. *Assessment of Future Scientific Needs for Live Variola Virus.* Washington, D.C.: National Academy Press, 1999.

Cronin, John, and Kennedy, Robert F., Jr. *The Riverkeepers: Two Activists Fight to Reclaim Our Environment as a Basic Human Right.* New York: Scribner, 1997.

Dando, Malcom. "Benefits and Threats of Developments in Biotechnology and Genetic Engineering." In *Stockholm International Peace Research Institute, Armaments, Disarmament, and International Security, 1999 Yearbook.* Oxford: Oxford University Press, 1999.

de Klemm, Cyrille. *Biological Diversity Conservation and the Law: Legal Mechanisms for Conserving Species and Ecosystems.* Gland, Switzerland: IUCN–the World Conservation Union, 1993.

DeSalle, Rob, ed. *Epidemic!: The World of Infectious Disease.* New York: New Press, 1999.

Ehrenfeld, David. *The Arrogance of Humanism.* New York: Oxford University Press, 1978.

Ehrlich, Paul, and Ehrlich, Anne. *Extinction: The Causes and Consequences of the Disappearance of Species.* New York: Random House, 1981.

Eldredge, Niles. *The Miner's Canary: Unraveling the Mysteries of Extinction.* New York: Prentice Hall, 1991.

Fenn, Elizabeth. *Pox Americana: The Great Smallpox Epidemic of 1775–82.* New York: Hill and Wang, 2001.

Fenner, Frank, Henderson, D. A., Arita, Isao, Jezek, Zdenek, and Ladnyi, Ivan D. *Smallpox and Its Eradication.* Geneva: World Health Organization, 1988.

Fischman, Robert L., and Squillace, Mark S. *Environmental Decisionmaking*, 3d ed. Cincinnati, Ohio: Anderson Publishing, 2000.

Fidler, David P. *International Law and Infectious Diseases.* New York: Oxford University Press, 1999.

Flowerree, Charles C. "Chemical and Biological Weapons and Arms Control." In ed. Richard Dean Burns, *Encyclopedia of Arms Control,* vol. 1. New York: Scribner's, 1993.

Garrett, Laurie. *Betrayal of Trust: The Collapse of Global Public Health.* New York: Hyperion, 2000.

Geissler, Erhard, ed. *Strengthening the Biological Weapons Convention by Confidence-Building Measures.* New York: Oxford University Press, 1990.

———, ed. *Biological and Toxin Weapons Today.* New York: Oxford University Press, 1986.

———. "Implications of Genetic Engineering for Chemical and Biological Warfare." In Stockholm International Peace Research Institute, *World Armaments and Disarmament, 1984 Yearbook.* Philadelphia: Taylor & Francis, 1984.

Geissler, Erhard, and Moon, John Ellis van Courtland, eds. *Biological and Toxin Weapons: Research, Development and Use from the Middle Ages to 1945.* New York: Oxford University Press, 1999.

Geissler, Erhard, and Woodall, John P., eds. *Control of Dual-Threat Agents: The Vaccines for Peace Programme.* New York: Oxford University Press, 1994.

Giblin, James Cross. *When Plague Strikes: The Black Death, Smallpox, AIDS.* New York: Harper Collins, 1995.

Guillemin, Jeanne. *Anthrax: The Investigation of a Deadly Outbreak.* Berkeley: University of California Press, 1999.

Guruswamy, Lakshman, and Hendricks, Brent. *International Environmental Law in a Nutshell.* St. Paul, Minn.: West Publishing, 1997.

Guruswamy, Lakshman D., Palmer, Geoffrey W. R., and Weston, Burns. *International Environmental Law and World Order.* St. Paul, Minn.: West Publishing, 1994.

Hamilton, Lawrence S., ed. *Ethics, Religion and Biodiversity: Relations between Conservation and Cultural Values.* Cambridge: White Horse Press, 1993.

Henderson, D. A. "Variola and Vaccinia." In ed. J. Claude Bennett and Fred Plum, *Cecil Textbook of Medicine,* 20th ed. Philadelphia: W.B. Saunders, 1996.

Hopkins, Donald R. *Princes and Peasants: Smallpox in History.* Chicago: University of Chicago Press, 1983.

Hunter, David, Salzman, James, and Zaelke, Durwood. *International Environmental Law and Policy.* New York: Foundation Press, 1998.

Hutton, Jon, and Dickson, Barnabas, eds. *Endangered Species, Threatened Convention: The Past, Present and Future of CITES.* London: Earthscan, 2000.

Innes, B. "Viruses." In *Encyclopedia of the Life Sciences,* vol. 10. Tarrytown, N.Y.: Marshall Cavendish Corp., 1996.

Johnson, George B., and Raven, Peter H. *Biology: Principles & Explorations.* Austin: Holt, Rinehart, and Winston, 1996.

Karlen, Arno. *Man and Microbes: Disease and Plagues in History and Modern Times.* New York: Simon & Schuster, 1995.

Mann, Charles C., and Plummer, Mark L. *Noah's Choice: The Future of Endangered Species.* New York: Knopf, 1996.

McCuen, Gary E., ed. *Biological Terrorism and Weapons of Mass Destruction.* Hudson, Wis.: G.E. McCuen Publications, 1999.

————, ed. *Poison in the Wind: The Spread of Chemical and Biological Weapons.* Hudson, Wis.: G.E. McCuen, 1992.

McInerney, Peter K., and Rainbolt, George W. *Ethics.* New York: HarperPerennial, 1994.

Moon, John Ellis van Courtland. "Controlling Chemical and Biological Weapons through World War II." In ed. Richard Dean Burns, *Encyclopedia of Arms Control,* vol. 1. New York: Scribner's, 1993.

Moya, Olga L., and Fono, Andrew L. *Federal Environmental Law: The User's Guide.* St. Paul, Minn.: West Publishing, 1997.

Norton, Bryan G., ed. *The Preservation of Species: The Value of Biological Diversity.* Princeton, N.J.: Princeton University Press, 1986.

Ogden, Horace G. *CDC and the Smallpox Crusade.* U.S. Department of Health and Human Services Publication No. (CDC) 87–8400. Washington, D.C.: U.S. GPO, 1987.

Oldstone, Michael B. A. *Viruses, Plagues, and History.* New York: Oxford University Press, 1998.

Parker, John. *The Killing Factory: The Top Secret World of Germ and Chemical Warfare.* London: Smith Gryphon, 1996.

Piller, Charles, and Yamamoto, Keith R. *Gene Wars: Military Control over the New Genetic Technologies.* New York: Beech Tree Books, 1988.

Reaka-Kudla, Marjorie L., Wilson, Don E., and Wilson, Edward O., eds. *Biodiversity II.* Washington, D.C.: Joseph Henry Press, 1997.

Regan, Tom. *The Case for Animal Rights.* Berkeley: University of California Press, 1983.

Regan, Tom, and Singer, Peter, eds. *Animal Rights and Human Obligations,* 2d ed. Englewood Cliffs, N.J.: Prentice Hall, 1989.

Regis, Ed. *Virus Ground Zero: Stalking the Killer Viruses with the Centers for Disease Control.* New York: Pocket Books, 1996.

Rogers, William H., Jr. *Environmental Law,* 2d ed. St. Paul, Minn.: West Publishing, 1994.

Rollin, Bernard E. *The Frankenstein Syndrome: Ethical and Social Issues in the Genetic Engineering of Animals.* New York: Cambridge University Press, 1995.

Schell, Jonathan. *The Fate of the Earth.* New York: Knopf, 1982.

Schiavone, Giuseppe. *International Organizations: A Directory and Dictionary*, 3d ed. New York: St. Martin's, 1993.

Scruton, Roger. *WHO, What and Why?: Trans-national Government, Legitimacy, and the World Health Organisation*. London: Institute of American Affairs, 2000.

Shurkin, Joel N. *The Invisible Fire: The Story of Mankind's Victory over the Ancient Scourge of Smallpox*. New York: Putnam, 1979.

Siddiqi, Javed. *World Health and World Politics: The World Health Organization and the UN System*. Columbia, S.C.: University of South Carolina Press, 1995.

Stearn, E. Wagner, and Stearn, Allen E. *The Effect of Smallpox on the Destiny of the Amerindian*. Boston: B. Humphries, 1945.

Steiner, Paul E. *Disease in the Civil War: Natural Biological Warfare in 1861–1865*. Springfield, Ill.: C.C. Thomas, 1968.

Stone, Christopher D. *Should Trees Have Standing and Other Essays on Law, Morals, and the Environment*. Dobbs Ferry, N.Y.: Oceana Publications, 1996.

———. *Earth and Other Ethics: The Case for Moral Pluralism*. New York: Harper & Row, 1987.

Swanson, Timothy. *Global Action for Diversity: An International Framework for Implementing the Convention on Biological Diversity*. London: Earthscan, 1997.

———. *The International Regulation of Extinction*. Washington Square: New York University Press, 1994.

Toward Mankind's Better Health. Study Guide Series, vol. 3. Dobbs Ferry, N.Y.: Oceana Publications, 1963.

Tucker, Jonathan B. *Scourge: The Once and Future Threat of Smallpox*. New York: Atlantic Monthly Press, 2001.

———, ed. *Toxic Terror: Assessing Terrorist Use of Chemical and Biological Weapons*. Cambridge, Mass.: MIT Press, 2000.

U.S. Arms Control and Disarmament Agency. *Arms Control and Disarmament Agreements: Texts and Histories of the Negotiations*. Washington, D.C.: U.S. Arms Control and Disarmament Agency, 1996.

Wells, Robert N., Jr., ed. *Peace by Pieces: United Nations Agencies and Their Roles*. Metuchen, N.J.: Scarecrow, 1991.

Weiss, Edith Brown. *In Fairness to Future Generations: International Law, Common Patrimony, and Intergenerational Equity*. Tokyo, Japan: United Nations University; Dobbs Ferry, N.Y.: Transnational Publishers, 1989.

Williams, Peter, and Wallace, David. *Unit 731: Japan's Secret Biological Warfare in World War II*. New York: Free Press, 1989.

Wilson, Edward O. *The Diversity of Life*. Cambridge, Mass.: Belknap Press of Harvard University Press, 1992.

Wise, Steven M. *Rattling the Cage: Toward Legal Rights for Animals.* Cambridge, Mass.: Perseus Books, 2000.

World Health Organization. *The First Ten Years of the World Health Organization.* Geneva: World Health Organization, 1958.

Worldmark Encyclopedia of the Nations: The United Nations, vol. 1, 10th ed. New York: Gale Research, 2001.

Wright, Susan, ed. *Preventing a Biological Arms Race.* Cambridge, Mass.: MIT Press, 1990.

Zanders, Jean Pascal, and Wahlberg, Maria. "Chemical and Biological Weapon Developments and Arms Control." In *SIPRI Yearbook 2000: Armaments, Disarmament, and International Security.* Stockholm: Almquist & Wiksell; New York: Humanities Press, 2000.

Articles and Reports

Adler, Jonathan H. "The Cartagena Protocol and Biological Diversity: Biosafe or Bio-Sorry?" *Georgetown International Environmental Law Review* 12, no. 3 (spring 2000), 761.

Advisory Committee on Immunization Practices. "Vaccinia (Smallpox) Vaccine Recommendations of the Advisory Committee on Immunization Practices." *MMWR Reports and Recommendations* 50, (June 22, 2001), 1–25.

Barquet, Nicolau, and Domingo, Pere. "Smallpox: The Triumph over the Most Terrible of the Ministers of Death." *Annals of Internal Medicine* 127 (October 15, 1997), 635.

Bernstein Barton J. "America's Biological Warfare Program in the Second World War." *Journal of Strategic Studies* (September 1988), 292.

Breman, Joel, and Henderson, D. A. "Poxvirus Dilemmas: Monkeypox, Smallpox, and Biologic Terrorism." *New England Journal of Medicine* 339, no. 8 (August 20, 1998), 556.

Capps, Linnea. "Smallpox and Biological Warfare: The Case for Abandoning Vaccination of Military Personnel." *American Journal of Public Health* 76, no. 10 (October 1986), 1229.

Center for Security Policy. "A Pox on *Our* House: Will Clinton's NSC Compound America's Vulnerability to Biological Warfare?" Decision Brief No. 99-D 36 (March 17, 1999).

Christensen, Eric. "Genetic Ark: A Proposal to Preserve Genetic Diversity for Future Generations." *Stanford Law Review* 40 (1987), 279.

Cigar, Norman. "Chemical Weapons and the Gulf War: The Dog That Did Not Bark." *Studies in Conflict and Terrorism* 15 (1992), 145.

Cohen, Jon. "Smallpox Vaccinations: How Much Protection Remains?" *Science* 294 (November 2, 2001), 985.

Dennis, Carina. "The Bugs of War." *Nature* 411 (May 17, 2001), 232.

Douglas, Joseph D., Jr. "The Challenges of Biochemical Warfare." *Global Affairs* 3 (1988), 156.

Dowdle, Walter R. "Destruction of the Smallpox Virus: Why the Debate?" *Clinical Microbiology Newsletter* 17, no. 13 (1995), 101.

Falk, Richard A. "Inhibiting Reliance on Biological Weaponry: The Role and Relevance of International Law." *American University Journal of International Law and Policy* 1 (1986), 17.

Feith, Douglas J. "Biological Weapons and the Limits of Arms Control." *National Interest* (winter 1986–1987), 80.

Fidler, David P. "The Return of 'Microbialpolitik.'" *Foreign Policy* (January/February 2001), 80.

———. "The Malevolent Use of Microbes and the Rule of Law: Legal Challenges Presented by Bioterrorism." *Clinical Infectious Diseases* 33 (2001), 636.

———. "The Future of the World Health Organization: What Role for International Law?" *Vanderbilt Journal of Transnational Law* 31, no. 5 (November 1998), 1079.

———. "Return of the Fourth Horseman: Emerging Infectious Diseases and International Law." *Minnesota Law Review* 81, no. 4 (April 1997), 771.

———. "Mission Impossible? International Law and Infectious Diseases." *Temple International & Comparative Law Journal* 10 (1996), 493.

Freedberg, Sydney J., Jr., and Serafini, Marilyn Werber. "Be Afraid, Be Moderately Afraid." *National Journal* (March 27, 1999), 806.

Friedmann, Theodore. "Overcoming the Obstacles to Gene Therapy." *Scientific American* (June 1997), 96.

Garrett, Laurie. "The Nightmare of Bioterrorism." *Foreign Affairs* 80, no. 1 (January/February 2001), 76.

———. "The Return of Infectious Disease." *Foreign Affairs* 75, no. 1 (January/February 1996), 66.

Gostin, Lawrence O., Burris, Scott, and Lazzarini, Zita. "The Law and the Public's Health: A Study of Infectious Disease Law in the United States." *Columbia Law Review* 99, no. 1 (January 1999), 59.

Harris, Elisa D. "Sverdlovsk and Yellow Rain: Two Cases of Soviet Noncompliance?" *International Security* 11, no. 4 (spring 1987), 41.

Henderson, D. A. "The Research Agenda Utilizing Variola Virus: A Public Health

Perspective." Working paper for WHO Committee Meeting on Smallpox (December 1999).

————. "Smallpox: Clinical and Epidemiologic Features." *Emerging Infectious Diseases* 5, no. 4 (July–August 1999), http://www.cdc.gov/ncidod/EID/vol5no4/henderson.htm, p. 2.

————. "Smallpox as a Biological Weapon: Medical and Public Health Management, Consensus Statement of the Working Group on Civilian Biodefense." *Journal of the American Medical Association* 281, no. 22 (June 9, 1999), 2127.

————. "Risk of a Deliberate Release of Smallpox Virus: Its Impact on Virus Destruction." Working Paper, Center for Civilian Biodefense Studies (January 1999).

————. "Deliberations Regarding the Destruction of Smallpox Virus: A Historical Overview, 1980–1998." Working paper for meeting of a Committee of the Institute of Medicine (November 20, 1998).

Henderson, D. A., and Fenner, Frank. "Recent Events and Observations Pertaining to Smallpox Virus Destruction in 2002." *Clinical Infectious Diseases* 33 (2001), 1057.

Joklik, Wolfgang K. "The Remaining Smallpox Virus Stocks Are Too Valuable to Be Destroyed." *The Scientist* (December 9, 1996), 11.

Joklik, Wolfgang K., Moss, Bernard, Fields, Bernard N., Bishop, David L., Sandakhchiev, Lev S. "Why the Smallpox Virus Stocks Should Not Be Destroyed." *Science* 262, no. 5137 (November 19, 1993).

Kreeger, Karen Young. "Smallpox Extermination Proposal Stirs Scientists." *The Scientist* 8, no. 22 (November 14, 1994), 1.

Langer, William L. "Immunization against Smallpox before Jenner." *Scientific American* 234, no. 1 (January 1976), 112.

LeDuc, James, and Becher, John. "Current Status of Smallpox Vaccine: Letter to the Editor." *Emerging Infectious Diseases* 5, no. 4 (July–August 1999), 593.

Mahy, Brian W. J., Almond, Jeffrey W., Berns, Kenneth I., Chanock, Robert M., Lvov, Dmitry K., Petterson, Ralf K., Schatzmeyer, Herman G., and Fenner, Frank. "The Remaining Stocks of Smallpox Should Be Destroyed." *Science* 262, no. 5137 (November 19, 1993).

Mann, Charles, and Plummer, Mark. "Is Endangered Species Act in Danger?" *Science* 267 (March 3, 1995), 1256.

McFarland, Stephen L. "Preparing for What Never Came: Chemical and Biological Warfare in World War II." *Brassey's Defense Analysis* 2 (1986), 107.

Meselson, Matthew. "Averting the Hostile Exploitation of Biotechnology." *CBW Conventions Bulletin* 48 (June 2000), 16.

Nagle, John Copeland. "Playing Noah." *Minnesota Law Review* 82, no. 5 (May 1998), 1171.

O'Toole, Tara. "Smallpox: An Attack Scenario." *Emerging Infectious Diseases* 5, no. 4 (July/August 1999), 540.

Orent, Wendy. "Killer Pox in the Congo." *Discover* 20, no. 10 (October 1999).

———. "The Smallpox Wars: Biowarfare vs Public Health." *American Prospect* 44 (May–June 1999), 49.

———. "Pox Populi." The Sciences 39, no. 1 (January/February 1999), 11.

———. "Escape from Moscow." *The Sciences* (May/June 1998), 26.

Parks, W. Hays. "Classification of Chemical-Biological Warfare." *Toledo Law Review* 13 (Summer 1982), 1165.

Pearson, Graham S. "Deliberate Disease: Why Biological Warfare is a Real Concern." International Security Information Service, Briefing Paper No. 6 (July 1996).

Piller, Charles. "Lethal Lies About Fatal Diseases." *The Nation* (October 3, 1988), 271.

Plotkin, Bruce Jay. "Mission Possible: The Future of the International Health Regulations." *Temple International & Comparative Law Journal* 10 (1986), 503.

Poupard, James A., Miller, Linda A., and Granshaw, Lindsay. "The Use of Smallpox as a Biological Weapon in the French and Indian War of 1763." *ASM News* 55, no. 3 (1989), 122.

Preston, Richard. "The Demon in the Freezer." *New Yorker* 75, no. 18 (July 12, 1999), 44.

Purver, Ron. "Chemical and Biological Terrorism: The Threat According to the Open Literature." *Canadian Security Intelligence Service* (June 1995).

Purvis, Andy, and Hector, Andy. "Getting the Measure of Biodiversity." *Nature* 405 (May 11, 2000), 212.

Radetsky, Michael. "Smallpox: A History of Its Rise and Fall." *Pediatric Infectious Disease Journal* 18, no. 2 (February 1999), 85.

Rimmington, Anthony. "From Military to Industrial Complex? The Conversion of Biological Weapons' Facilities in the Russian Federation." *Contemporary Security Policy* 17, no. 1 (April 1996), 80.

Roizman, Bernard, Joklik, Wolfgang, Fields, Bernard, and Moss, Bernard. "The Destruction of Smallpox Virus Stocks in National Repositories: A Grave Mistake and a Bad Precedent." *Infectious Agents and Disease* 3, no. 5 (1994), 215.

Sandakhchiev, Lev S. "We'd Better Think Twice Before Eradicating All Smallpox Virus Stocks." *The Scientist* 7, no. 16 (August 23, 1993), 11.

Serafini, Marilyn Werber. "A New Smallpox Vaccine: How Safe?" *National Journal* (October 27, 2001), 3371.

Taylor, Allyn L. "Controlling the Global Spread of Infectious Diseases: Toward a Reinforced Role for the International Health Regulations." *Houston Law Review* 33 (1997), 1327.

―――. "Making the World Health Organization Work: A Legal Framework for Universal Access to the Conditions for Health." *American Journal of Law & Medicine* 18, no. 4 (1992), 301.

Thranert, Oliver. "Strengthening the Biological Weapons Convention: An Urgent Task." *Contemporary Security Policy* 17, no. 3 (December 1996), 347.

Toulmin, Stephen. "The Case for Cosmic Prudence." *Tennessee Law Review* 56 (1988), 29.

Tucker, Jonathan B. "Biological Weapons in the Former Soviet Union: An Interview with Dr. Kenneth Alibek." *Nonproliferation Review* 6, no. 3 (spring–summer 1999), 1.

―――. "Gene Wars." *Foreign Policy* (winter 1984), 58.

U.S. Central Intelligence Agency. "The Global Infectious Disease Threat and Its Implications for the United States." National Intelligence Estimate 99-17D (January 2000), 16.

U.S. Government. "Report on Activities and Programs for Countering Proliferation and NBC Terrorism." Counterproliferation Program Review Committee (May 1998).

Venter, Al J. "Sverdlovsk Outbreak: A Portent of Disaster." *Jane's Intelligence Review* 10, no. 5 (May 1, 1998), 36.

World Health Organization. "Report by the Secretariat: Smallpox Eradication Temporary Retention of Variola Virus Stocks." A54/16, April 11, 2001, 2.

―――. "Report by the Secretariat: Smallpox Eradication: Destruction of Variola Virus Stocks." April 10, 2000, EB 106/3.

―――. "Overcoming Antimicrobial Resistance." World Health Report on Infectious Diseases (2000).

World Health Organization, Department of Communicable Disease Surveillance and Response. "WHO Advisory Committee on Variola Virus Research: Report of a WHO Meeting, Geneva, Switzerland, 6–9 December 1999." WHO/CDS/CSR/2000.1

―――. "Report of the meeting of the Ad Hoc Committee on Orthopoxvirus Infections." Geneva, Switzerland, January 14–15, 1999, WHO/CDS/CSR/99.1.

Wright, Susan. "The Buildup That Was." *Bulletin of the Atomic Scientists* (January/February) 1989, 52.

Newspaper Articles

Altman, Lawrence K. "Plan for Smallpox Rules Out Mass Vaccination," *New York Times*, November 27, 2001, B7.

———. "U.S. Sets Up Plan to Fight Smallpox in Case of Attack." *New York Times*, November 4, 2001, A1.

———. "Fate of a Virus: A Special Report." *New York Times*, August 30, 1993, A1.

Altman, Lawrence K., Broad, William J., and Miller, Judith. "Smallpox: The Once and Future Scourge?" *New York Times*, June 15, 1999, F1.

Angier, Natalie. "Defining the Undefinable: Being Alive." *New York Times*, December 18, 2001, D1.

Bradsher, Keith. "3 Smaller Companies Say Their Vaccines Are Cheaper." *New York Times*, November 8, 2001, B9.

———. "U.S. Begins Search for Medicine Used to Treat Adverse Reactions to Smallpox Vaccine." *New York Times*, October 22, 2001, B9.

Broad, William J., and Miller, Judith. "Government Report Says 3 Nations Hide Stocks of Smallpox." *New York Times*, June 13, 1999, A1.

———. "Germ Defense Plan in Peril as Its Flaws Are Revealed." *New York Times*, August 7, 1998, A1.

Brown, David. "U.S. Wants the Smallpox Virus Preserved for Further Research." *Washington Post*, November 17, 2001, A9.

Brownlee, Shannon. "Clear and Present Danger." *Washington Post Magazine*, October 28, 2001, 8.

Connolly, Ceci. "Some Want Smallpox Shots Now." *Washington Post*, December 26, 2001, A1.

Connolly, Ceci, and Gillis, Justin. "U.S. to Buy Smallpox Vaccine." *Washington Post*, November 29, 2001, A10.

Ewald, Paul W. "A Risky Policy on Smallpox Vaccinations." *New York Times*, December 17, 2001, A23.

Gillis, Justin. "U.S. Limits Bids on Vaccines." *Washington Post*, November 11, 2001, A14.

Kucewicz, William. "Beyond Yellow Rain: The Threat of Soviet Genetic Engineering." *Wall Street Journal*, April 23–May 18, 1984.

Kolata, Gina. " 'Cure' for Bioterror May Be Worse Than the Disease." *New York Times*, October 22, 2001, B9.

Miller, Judith. "U.S. Set to Retain Smallpox Stocks." *New York Times*, November 16, 2001, A1.

Miller, Judith, and Stolberg, Sheryl Gay. "Attacks Led to Push for More Smallpox Vaccine." *New York Times*, October 22, 2001, A1.

Okie, Susan. "Preparing for Invisible Killers: Smallpox and Anthrax Could Be Put to Work in Biological Warfare." *Washington Post,* February 23, 1999, Health Section, 7.

Okie, Susan, and Gillis, Justin. "U.S. Mounts Smallpox Vaccine Push." *Washington Post,* October 28, 2001, A18.

Orent, Wendy. "The End of the Trail for Smallpox?" *Los Angeles Times,* August 2, 1998, M2.

Pianin, Eric, and Nakashima, Ellen. "U.S. Seeks to Boost Security, Soothe Public." *Washington Post,* October 18, 2001, A1.

Siebert, Charles. "Smallpox Is Dead, Long Live Smallpox." *New York Times Magazine,* August 21, 1994, 30.

Stolberg, Sheryl Gay. "Some Experts Say U.S. Is Vulnerable to a Germ Attack." *New York Times,* September 30, 2001, A1.

Stolberg, Sheryl Gay, and Miller, Judith. "Bioterror Role an Uneasy Fit for the C.D.C." *New York Times,* November 11, 2001, A1.

Stolberg, Sheryl Gay, with Petersen, Melody. "U.S. Orders Vast Supply of Vaccine for Smallpox." *New York Times,* November 29, 2001, B8.

Thatcher, Gary. "Disease as an Agent of War." *Christian Science Monitor Special Report,* December 15, 1988, B4.

Weiss, Rick. "Genetic Find Could Lead to Creation of Life From Scratch in Lab." *Washington Post,* December 10, 1999, A8.

Yoon, Carol Kaesuk. "If It Walks and Moos Like a Cow, It's a Pharmaceutical Factory." *New York Times,* May 1, 2000, A20.

Index

accidents in laboratories or testing facilities, 7, 25–26, 42, 55, 69, 79–80, 182–84, 224

Ad Hoc Committee on Orthopox Virus Infections, 146–47, 154, 214

Advisory Committee on Variola Virus Research, 148, 150–51

African Convention on Conservation of Nature and Natural Resources, 118

alastrim, 16

Alexander the Great, 11, 59

Alibek, Ken, 72, 87

amaas, 16

Amherst, Sir Jeffrey, 62, 190

anthrax: in Iraqi weapons program, 84–85; and October 2001 attacks, 28, 90–91, 97, 152–53, 209; as potential biological warfare agent, 50, 58, 59, 74, 209; and Soviet accident at Sverdlovsk, 79–80, 184; in Soviet Union research program, 71–73; stockpiling and use of during World War II, 66–69; terrorist use or attempted use of, 95–98, 152; use of during World War I, 64

Ashcroft, John, 99

Aum Shinrikyo, 95–96

Australia Group, 73–74

autoclave, 2, 126, 128, 147, 154, 166, 187, 191, 200, 206, 227

Aventis Pasteur, 28

Aztecs, 13, 61

Bedson, Harry, 26

Bernard, Ken, 49

bifurcated needle, 22, 27, 217

biodiversity, *see* biological diversity

Biodiversity Convention, 115–18, 124, 194, 210

biological agents, 73–76, 130; and cold war programs, 68–70; genetic engineering of, 41–42, 86–88, 191; history of use, 3–4, 58–63, 190–91; proliferation, 83–86; in Soviet Union programs, 71–73, 79–83, 180, 184, 199, 207, 215, 225; and terrorist threat, 88–99, 201, 212, 219–20; treaties to regulate, 64–65, 76–81, 99–101, 170, 190–92, 221; in twentieth-century programs, 64–68; in warfare and weapons, 47, 50, 152, 168, 185, 202, 206, 211, 213, 216

biological dimension, 3, 32–57, 208

259

Project Coordinator:	Green Sand Press, Tucson
Compositor:	BookMatters, Berkeley
Text:	9.75/15 Minion
Display:	Cholla Unicase and Conduit ITC Light
Printer and Binder:	Maple-Vail Manufacturing Group

ALTHOUGH SMALLPOX WAS OFFICIALLY ERADICATED FROM THE PLANET TWENTY YEARS AGO,

recent terrorist acts have raised the horrific possibility that rogue states, laboratories, or terrorist groups are in possession of secret stockpiles of the virus that causes the disease and may be preparing to unleash it on target populations. Because it is far deadlier than other biological warfare agents such as anthrax, and because universal vaccination against smallpox was halted decades ago, a smallpox attack today would be nothing short of catastrophic. This clear, authoritative study looks at the long and fascinating history of the virus, with an examination of the political, biological, environmental, medical, and legal issues surrounding the question of whether the remaining known stocks of the virus should be destroyed.

The only two known samples of the virus are currently stored in Atlanta and in Novosibirsk, Russia. The World Health Organization has repeatedly scheduled (and postponed) their destruction—an action that would rid the planet of all publicly acknowledged smallpox strains forever. Opponents of this plan argue that destroying these last samples is to deny the possibility that this unique virus

3663